# Essentials of Pharmacology

Custom Version for Renton Technical College

Ruth Woodrow / Bruce Colbert / David Smith

CENGAGE
Learning·

Australia • Brazil • Japan • Korea • Mexico • Singapore • Spain • United Kingdom • United States

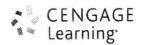

**Essentials of Pharmacology
Custom Version for Renton Technical
College**

Senior Manager, Student Engagement:
Linda deStefano

Manager, Student Engagement:
Julie Dierig

Manager, Student Engagement:
Janey Moeller

Senior Marketing Manager:
Heather Kramer

Manager, Production Editorial:
Kim Fry

Manager, Intellectual Property Project Manager:
Brian Methe

Senior Manager, Production and Manufacturing:
Donna M. Brown

Manager, Production:
Terri Daley

Essentials of Pharmacology for Health Professions, Seventh Edition
Woodrow/Colbert/Smith
© 2015, 2011, 2007, 2002 Cengage Learning. All rights reserved.

For product information and technology assistance, contact us at
**Cengage Learning Customer & Sales Support, 1-800-354-9706**

For permission to use material from this text or product,
submit all requests online at **cengage.com/permissions**
Further permissions questions can be emailed to
**permissionrequest@cengage.com**

This book contains select works from existing Cengage Learning resources and
was produced by Cengage Learning Custom Solutions for collegiate use. As such,
those adopting and/or contributing to this work are responsible for editorial
content accuracy, continuity and completeness.

**Compilation © 2014Cengage Learning**

ISBN-13: 978-1-305-28709-9

ISBN-10: 1-305-28709-6

**WCN: 01-100-101**

**Cengage Learning**
5191 Natorp Boulevard
Mason, Ohio 45040
USA
Cengage Learning is a leading provider of customized learning solutions with
office locations around the globe, including Singapore, the United Kingdom,
Australia, Mexico, Brazil, and Japan. Locate your local office at:
**international.cengage.com/region.**

Cengage Learning products are represented in Canada by Nelson Education, Ltd.
For your lifelong learning solutions, visit **www.cengage.com/custom.**
Visit our corporate website at **www.cengage.com.**

Printed in the United States of America

# Brief Contents

# CHAPTER 2

## DRUG NAMES AND REFERENCES

## Objectives

*Upon completion of this chapter, the learner should be able to*

1. Describe drug classification systems
2. Differentiate among the following drug names: generic name, official name, trade name, and chemical name
3. Explain what is indicated by a number included in a drug trade name (e.g., Tylenol No. 3)
4. Contrast generic and brand name drugs
5. Define and explain the restrictions of drug sales implied by the following: OTC, legend drug, and controlled substance
6. Discuss the various terms indicating drug actions contained in reference sources
7. List and describe at least two drug references available today
8. Discuss several characteristics that you consider important in choosing the best drug reference
9. Describe how to evaluate drug information websites
10. Define the Key Terms and Concepts

## Key Terms and Concepts

Actions
Adverse reactions
Cautions
Classifications
Contraindications
Generic names
Indications
Interactions
Legend drug
Official name
Pharmacology
Prototype
Side effects
Trade names

Pharmacology can be defined as the study of drugs and their origin, nature, properties, and effects on living organisms. We need to know why drugs are given, how they work, and what effects to expect. The thousands of drug products on the market would make this subject difficult to tackle if it were not for:

- Numerous drug references, geared to a variety of levels of readers, from layperson to pharmacist
- Grouping of drugs under broad subcategories
- Continuity in the use of basic identifying terms for the names and actions of drugs

# CLASSIFICATIONS

Each drug can be categorized under a broad *subcategory,* or *subcategories,* called classifications. While drugs can be classified in several different ways, grouping them together according to their therapeutic use is most helpful to the health care professional. Drugs that affect the body in similar ways are listed in the same classification. Drugs that have several types of therapeutic effects fit under several classifications. For example, aspirin has a variety of effects on the body. It may be given to relieve pain (analgesic), to reduce fever (antipyretic), to reduce inflammation of tissues (anti-inflammatory), or as an anti-platelet (anti-thrombotic agent). Therefore, aspirin is categorized under four classifications of drugs (as shown in parentheses).

Another drug, cyclobenzaprine (Flexeril), however, is known to be used for only one therapeutic effect: to relieve muscle spasms. Flexeril, therefore, is listed only under the one classification of muscle relaxant.

Examples of some common drug classifications are listed in Table 2-1. Are you familiar with any of them already?

The second part of this text compares the characteristics of the various major drug classifications. In each chapter, as a classification is explained, you will learn what general information to associate with drugs of that classification, including:

- Therapeutic uses
- Most common side effects
- Precautions to be used
- Contraindications (when *not* to use the drug)
- Interactions that may occur when taken with other drugs or foods
- Some of the most common product names, usual dosages, and comments on administration

You may also be given a prototype of each classification. A prototype is a *model example,* a drug that typifies the characteristics of that classification. For example, propranolol (Inderal) is the prototype of the beta-adrenergic blockers (see Chapter 13).

**TABLE 2-1** Examples of Common Drug Classifications

| CLASSIFICATION | THERAPEUTIC USE | DRUG EXAMPLE(S) |
|---|---|---|
| Analgesic | Relieves pain without loss of consciousness | ibuprofen, aspirin, Tylenol |
| Antacid | Neutralizes stomach acid | Mylanta, Maalox |
| Anticoagulant | Prevents or delays blood clotting | heparin, Coumadin |
| Antianxiety | Reduces anxiety | Valium, Xanax |
| Antitussive | Prevents or relieves cough | codeine |
| Diuretic | Increases urinary output | Lasix |
| Hypoglycemic | Reduces blood glucose (sugar) levels | insulin |

Hopefully, each time you learn of a new drug, you will associate the prototype and its characteristics with the new drug, based on its classification.

You can find the classification as well as the various names of a drug by referring to a drug reference source.

# IDENTIFYING NAMES

Drug names can seem very complicated because a single drug will have many names attached to it. Four specific names can apply to each approved drug:

1. ***Generic name.***
   a. Common or general name assigned to the drug by the United States Adopted Name (USAN) Council
   b. Differentiated from the trade name by initial lowercase letter
   c. Never capitalized
2. ***Trade name.***
   a. The name by which a pharmaceutical company identifies its product
   b. Copyrighted and used exclusively by that company
   c. Distinguished from the generic name by capitalized first letter
   d. Often shown on labels and references with the symbol ® after the name (for "registered" trademark)
3. ***Chemical name.***
   a. The exact molecular formula of the drug
   b. Usually a long, very difficult name to pronounce
   c. Of little concern to the health care practitioner
4. ***Official name.***
   a. Name of the drug as it appears in the official reference, the USP/NF
   b. Generally the same as the generic name

The use of generic names and trade names for drugs can be compared to the various names of grocery products. Two examples of generic names are orange juice and detergent. Corresponding trade names for orange juice are Sunkist, Bird's Eye, Tropicana, and Minute Maid, while Cheer, Tide, All, and Fab are trade names for detergents. While there is only one generic name, there may be many trade names.

When a company produces a new drug for the market, it assigns a generic name to the product. After testing and approval by the FDA, the drug company gives the drug a trade name (often something short and easy to remember when advertised). For five years, from the time the company submits a *new drug application (NDA)* to the FDA for approval, the company has the exclusive right to market the drug. Once approved, the drug is listed in the USP/NF by an official name, which is usually the same as the generic name. After five years have passed and the patent has expired (although patent extensions are requested and frequently granted), other companies may begin to combine the same chemicals to form that specific generic product for marketing. Each company will assign its own specific trade name to the product, or the drug can be offered simply by its generic name and strength, such as acetaminophen 325 mg. See Table 2-2, which compares the names for two drugs.

**TABLE 2-2** Comparison of Drug Names

| GENERIC NAME | CHEMICAL NAME | TRADE NAMES (DRUG COMPANY) |
|---|---|---|
| doxycycline hyclate | 2-Naphthacenecarboxamide, 4-(dimethylamino)-1,4,4a,5,5a,6,11,12a-octahydro-3,5,10,12,12a-pentahydroxy-6-methyl-1,11-dioxo-, (4S,4aR,5S,5aR, 6R,12aS)-(564-25-0) | Vibramycin (PD-RX Pharmaceuticals) doxycycline hyclate[a] (West-Ward) |
| chlordiazepoxide hydrochloride | 7-chloro-2 methylamino-5 phenyl-3H-1,4-benzodiazephine 4-oxide hydrochloride | Librium |

[a] Some companies simply elect to market the product by the generic name.

# PATIENT EDUCATION

Patients may ask you about the difference between generic and trade (brand) name products. The FDA regulates the manufacturing of generic drugs, so patients can be assured they are safe and cost-effective alternatives. Generally, trade name products are more expensive, although the basic active ingredients (drug contents) are the same as those in the generic. The higher price helps to pay for the costs of drug development and advertisements promoting the trade name. (Can you think of certain trade names that are heavily advertised in television commercials?)

Since generic drug equivalents may exist for both prescription and over-the-counter (OTC) drug products, it is often economically wise to check for medicines that have the same generic components and strengths. For example, several cough syrups may have exactly the same contents, but the prices may vary widely.

Read and compare all ingredients on the labels.

Concerning prescription drugs, most states have enacted legislation encouraging physicians to let pharmacists substitute less expensive *generic equivalents* for prescribed brand name drugs. Specific provisions of drug *substitution laws* vary from state to state.

The physician may indicate "no substitutions" on the prescription, usually indicated by a *dispense as written (DAW) order*. Often physicians have preferences for certain products or patients may be difficult to stabilize on a certain class of medications (such as thyroid preparations). Even though the drug contents are the same, the "fillers," or ingredients that are used to hold the preparation together, may be slightly different. This difference in fillers may affect how quickly the drug dissolves or takes effect. Dyes in some products may alter effects in some sensitive patients by leading to an allergic response.

Many products are combinations of several generic components. You will recognize this when you see several generic names (not capitalized) and their corresponding amounts listed under one trade name (capitalized). Examples are given in Table 2-3.

| **TABLE 2-3** Examples of Combination Drugs | |
|---|---|
| **TRADE NAME** | **GENERIC NAME AND AMOUNT** |
| Dyazide (used to treat high blood pressure) | hydrochlorothiazide 25 mg, triamterene 37.5 mg |
| Glucovance (used to treat Type 2 diabetes mellitus) | glyburide 1.25 mg, metformin 250 mg<br>glyburide 2.5 mg, metformin 500 mg<br>glyburide 5 mg, metformin 500 mg |
| Robitussin DM 5 mL syrup | dextromethorphan, 10 mg; guaifenesin, 100 mg |

It should be noted that a number may be part of the trade name. The number often refers to an amount of one of the generic components and helps to differentiate it from an almost identical product. Identify the significance of the numbers in comparing the following trade names:

| Trade Name | Generic Name and Amount |
|---|---|
| Tylenol No. 2 | acetaminophen 300 mg codeine 15 mg |
| Tylenol No. 3 | acetaminophen 300 mg codeine 30 mg |
| Tylenol No. 4 | acetaminophen 300 mg codeine 60 mg |

Note that each product contains the same amount of acetaminophen, with varying amounts of the controlled substance codeine. *The larger the number in the name, the greater is the amount of controlled substance present.*

Many drug errors have occurred because the trade name was misinterpreted for the number of tablets to be given. So . . .

> **Be certain you can clearly read and understand the order!**

Another type of drug error involves preventable allergic reactions to one of the generic components of a medication. The problem stems from:

- Not consulting the patient's chart for the history of allergies before a new medication is ordered or given
- Not checking a reference to find out if a medication being ordered or given contains any generic components to which the patient has a known allergy

For example, if a patient has an allergy to aspirin, do not administer the first dose of any new medication to the patient without finding out if the product contains aspirin. Although the physician is in error for ordering the medication, you are also in error for administering a medication with which you are unfamiliar. A proficient health care practitioner should check the history and chart for known allergies and pick up any discrepancies. Alertness is the key to safety in any setting.

According to the Institute for Safe Medication Practices (ISMP) and the Food and Drug Administration (FDA), look-alike and sound-alike medications are a leading cause of drug errors. For example, the generic drug clonidine used for high blood pressure can be confused with the brand name drug Klonopin used for seizures; Celebrex for arthritis can be confused with Celexa for depression.

These two agencies have created a long-standing relationship with a goal of preventing drug errors. The ISMP has developed tools such as the "List of Confused Drug Names" as a quick drug reference that is available on its website at http://www.ismp.org.

> Always keep a drug reference handy, and use it when you are unfamiliar with the generic components of a drug ordered for a patient with known drug allergies. With experience, you will learn and remember the names of products most commonly used at your facility.

## LEGAL TERMS REFERRING TO DRUGS

A drug may be referred to by terms other than its classification, generic name, trade name, chemical name, or official name. As mentioned in Chapter 1, the following terms imply the legal accessibility of a drug:

1. *Over-the-counter (OTC) drug.* No purchasing restrictions by the FDA (with some exceptions, such as pseudoephedrine, which is OTC, but kept behind the pharmacy counter; see Chapter 20)

2. *Legend drug.* Prescription drug; determined unsafe for OTC purchase because of possible harmful side effects if taken indiscriminately; includes birth control pills, antibiotics, cardiac drugs, and hormones

3. *Controlled substance.* Drug controlled by prescription requirement because of the danger of addiction or abuse; indicated in references by schedule numbers C-I to C-V (see Chapter 1)

> The legend drug is so named because it requires a legend or warning statement that says, "Federal law prohibits dispensing without a prescription."

Figure 2-1 shows the information contained on a drug label including the trade name (Percocet) and the generic names of the two drugs (oxycodone and acetaminophen) that it contains. In addition, can you find the controlled substance marking?

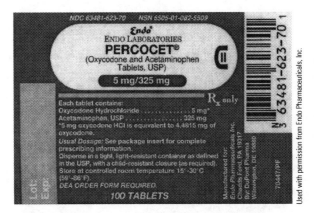

Used with permission from Endo Pharmaceuticals, Inc.

**FIGURE 2-1** Information contained on a drug label including the trade name (Percocet) and the generic names of the two drugs (oxycodone and acetaminophen) that it contains.

# TERMS INDICATING DRUG ACTIONS

Most references follow a similar format in describing drugs. When you research drug information, you will find the following terms as headings under each drug. You will find specific information more quickly if you understand what is listed under each heading.

*Indications.* A list of medical conditions or diseases for which the drug is meant to be used (e.g., diphenhydramine hydrochloride [Benadryl] is a commonly used drug; indications include allergic rhinitis, mild allergic skin reactions, motion sickness, and mild cases of parkinsonism).

*Actions.* A description of the cellular changes that occur as a result of the drug. This information tends to be very technical, describing cellular and tissue changes. While it is helpful to know what body system is affected by the drug, this information is geared more for the pharmacist (e.g., as an antihistamine, Benadryl appears to compete with histamine for cell receptor sites on effector cells).

*Contraindications.* A list of conditions for which the drug should *not* be given (e.g., two common contraindications for Benadryl are breast-feeding and hypersensitivity).

*Cautions.* A list of conditions or types of patients that warrant closer observation for specific side effects when given the drug (e.g., due to atropine-like activity, Benadryl must be used cautiously with patients who have a history of bronchial asthma or glaucoma, or with older adults [see Chapter 27]).

*Side effects and adverse reactions.* A list of possible unpleasant or dangerous secondary effects, other than the desired effect (e.g., side effects of Benadryl include sedation, dizziness, disturbed coordination, epigastric distress, anorexia, and thickening of bronchial secretions). This listing may be quite extensive, with as many as 50 or more side effects for one drug. Because it is difficult to know which are most likely to occur, choose a reference that highlights the most common side effects. Certain drugs may have side effects with which you are not familiar. Note the definitions of the following three side effects associated with specific antibiotics.

- Ototoxicity causes damage to the eighth cranial nerve, resulting in impaired hearing or ringing in the ears (tinnitus). Damage may be reversible or permanent.
- Nephrotoxicity causes damage to the kidneys, resulting in impaired kidney function, decreased urinary output, and renal failure.
- Photosensitivity is an increased reaction to sunlight, with the danger of intense sunburn.

*Interactions.* A list of other drugs or foods that may alter the effect of the drug and usually should not be given during the same course of therapy (e.g., monoamine oxidase [MAO] inhibitors will intensify the effects of Benadryl; you will find MAO inhibitors listed under interactions for many drugs; the term refers to a group of drugs that have been used for the treatment of depression; it has been found that they can cause serious blood pressure changes, and even death, when taken with many other drugs and some foods).

Other headings often listed under information about a drug include "How Supplied" and "Usual Dosage." "How Supplied" lists the available forms and strengths of the drug. "Usual Dosage" lists the amount of drug considered safe for administration, the route, and the frequency of administration. For example:

How supplied: tablets (tabs): 20 mg and 40 mg; suppository: 20 mg

Usual dosage: 10 mg orally every 4 h (q4h)

For a listing of common abbreviations regarding drug administration and medication orders, see Tables 4-1 and 5-1 in the upcoming chapters.

# DRUG REFERENCES

*Physicians' Desk Reference (PDR)* is one of the most widely used references for drugs in current use. It is available online, as a mobile app, and in book form. There are three versions of the *PDR*, one for physicians, one for nurses, and one for consumers. In addition, there are many new choices of references available today. Three are compared here, including the *PDR*. You must find the reference most suitable for you, one that you can interpret quickly and easily. By becoming knowledgeable about the drugs you administer, you may prevent possible drug errors from occurring.

Physician's Desk Reference (PDR)*

| PRO | CON |
|---|---|
| 1. *PDR* for Physicians—Available for free online, as a mobile app, and for a fee in book form. Benefits include: | Contains only those drugs that manufacturers pay to have incorporated |
|   Product labeling | Incomplete with regard to OTC drugs, making it necessary to buy *PDR* OTC book |
|   FDA drug safety communication | |
|   Medication guide | |
|   Drug alerts, recalls, and approvals | |
|   Patient resources | |
|   Various tools such as e-Books and mobile *PDR* | |
|   Ability to report of adverse reactions | |
|   Photographs of many drugs for product identification | |
| 2. *PDR* for Nurses—available for a fee Free mobile apps | |
|   Includes 1,500 FDA-regulated drugs | |
|   Includes critical black box warnings | |
| 3. *PDR* for Consumers—written in patient-friendly language | |
|   Includes over 300 prescribed drugs | |
|   Color images of medications | |
|   Comparison tables of OTC drugs | |
|   Guide to safe medication use | |

*Published annually by PDR Network, LLC, Montvale, New Jersey.

United States Pharmacopeia and the National Formulary (USP.NF)†

| PRO | CON |
|---|---|
| Information is available online at http://www.usp.org | No photographs of drugs |
| Provides information on and standards for chemical and biological drug substances, dosage forms, and compounded preparations; medical devices; and dietary supplements. | Geared for laboratory and manufacturing use |
| | No easily identified nursing implications |
| | Can be confusing to use |

†Published annually by U.S. Pharmacopeial Convention, Inc., Rockville, Maryland.

AHFS Drug Information (American Health-System Formulary Service)‡

| PRO | CON |
|---|---|
| Distributed to practicing physicians; single paperback volume, includes mobile drug reference and handbook to injectable drugs | Some parts (e.g., "Chemical Information" and "Drug Stability") not necessary for the health care practitioner |
| Good, concise information; easy to read | No photographs of drugs |
| Arranged by classifications, with a general statement about each classification at the beginning of each section | |
| Off-label drug indications are listed (not FDA approved) http://www.ashp.org/ | |

‡Published annually by American Society of Health-System Pharmacists, Bethesda, Maryland.

Other references (e.g., *The Pill Book, Handbook of Nonprescription Drugs*) may be found in bookstores, but they may not contain adequate information for the health care practitioner. Your school may recommend a specific drug reference other than the three listed in this text. Many new references geared to the nurse or health care practitioner are currently being published. Electronic drug references such as Lexi-Drugs and/or Epocrates (a free version of this) are also widely used.

# THE INTERNET AS REFERENCE

The Internet offers a wealth of information regarding medications and the conditions they treat. However, there can be serious dangers associated with some online sources that may not be reliable, professional, or even legitimate. Therefore, care must be taken to identify and use only websites that are supervised and controlled, such as those under the auspices of government agencies or sponsored by professional pharmacist groups. It is important for the health care practitioner to obtain accurate information and also be able to direct the patient or client to reliable sources of information regarding medicines. It is the health care practitioner's responsibility to caution the layperson regarding the controversial and dangerous practices of "online prescribing" without ever evaluating the patient in person, or obtaining medicines without prescriptions through the Internet.

| **EVALUATING INTERNET DRUG SOURCES** | Remember that all websites are not created equal. Pay attention to a few simple rules when seeking the most reputable ones. <br><br> 1. Check the source. Have scientific studies been done with a large enough sample? Are results reliable and valid? Are there links to a page listing professional credentials or affiliations? <br> 2. Check the date of articles. Medicine is a rapidly evolving field. Information can go out of date quickly. <br> 3. Be wary of information from forums and testimonials. Motivations are unknown. The information is not necessarily valid, and there may be a hidden agenda. |
|---|---|

The following websites are reliable professional sources of medical information:

| | |
|---|---|
| http://www.pharmacist.com | Sponsored by the American Pharmacists Association (APhA), the national professional society of pharmacists. |
| http://www.fda.gov | U.S. Food and Drug Administration, includes "Human Drugs" and Center for Drug Evaluation and Research (CDER). |
| http://www.safemedication.com | Sponsored by the American Society of Health-System Pharmacists. Covers correct dosage, side effects, and optimal use of most prescriptions and OTC drugs. Also offers reports on topics such as antibiotic-resistant bacteria. |

| | |
|---|---|
| http://www.usp.org | U.S. Pharmacopeial Convention (USP/DI) (See United States Pharmacopeia, previous page. |
| http://www.cdc.gov/vaccines/ | U.S. Centers for Disease Control and Prevention, National Immunization Program. Covers vaccines and immunizations. |
| http://www.nlm.nih.gov/medlineplus/ | A service of the U.S. National Library of Medicine and the National Institutes of Health. A great source for medicine and related health topics. |

# CHAPTER REVIEW QUIZ

**Match the definition with the term.**

1. _____ List of conditions for which a drug is meant to be used
2. _____ Subcategories of drugs based on their effects on the body
3. _____ Description of the cellular changes that occur as a result of a drug
4. _____ Conditions for which a drug should not be given

    **a.** Contraindications
    **b.** Precautions
    **c.** Indications
    **d.** Prototype
    **e.** Actions
    **f.** Classifications

**Refer to the following drug description to answer questions 5–8.**

AZO Standard®
(phenazopyridine HCl tablets, USP)
Product of i-Health, a Division of DSM
Description: AZO Standard (phenazopyridine HCl) is a urinary tract analgesic agent, chemically designated 2,6-pyridinediamine, 3-(phenylazo), monohydrochloride.

5. The generic name of the drug is _____.
6. The chemical name of the drug is _____.
7. The trade name of the drug is _____.
8. What is indicated by the ® symbol after the drug name?

_____

9. List three drug references:

_____

_____

_____

10. Explain the difference between these two medication orders:
    **a.** Give two Tylenol, PO.
    **b.** Give one Tylenol No #2 PO.

_____

_____

11. An older adult male was found unconscious in his bedroom with several pink and blue pills beside his bed, but no labeled pill bottle can be found. He is rushed to the emergency department for treatment. What drug reference source will be most helpful in this situation?

_____

---

**STUDY**GUIDE

**P R A C T I C E**

Complete Chapter 2

**Online Resources**LINK

• PowerPoint presentations

# CHAPTER 7

## RESPONSIBILITIES AND PRINCIPLES OF DRUG ADMINISTRATION

## Objectives

*Upon completion of this chapter, the learner should be able to*

1. Describe four responsibilities of the health care provider in safe administration of medications
2. List the six Rights of Medication Administration
3. Explain moral, ethical, and legal responsibilities regarding medication errors
4. Cite three instances of medication administration that require documentation
5. Explain the rights of the health care practitioner to question or refuse to administer medications
6. Define the Key Terms and Concepts

## Key Terms and Concepts

Documentation of drug administration

Medication Errors Reporting (MER) program

Medication reconciliation

Reporting of medication errors

Responsibilities of drug administration

Six Rights of Medication Administration

MedWatch

## RESPONSIBLE DRUG ADMINISTRATION

The safe and accurate administration of medications requires knowledge, judgment, and skill. The responsibilities of the health care provider in this vital area include:

1. Adequate, up-to-date *information* about all medications to be administered, including their purpose, potential side effects, cautions and contraindications, and possible interactions.

2. *Wisdom* and judgment to accurately *assess* the patient's needs for medications, to *evaluate* the response to medications, and to *plan* appropriate interventions as indicated.

3. *Skill in delivery* of the medication accurately, in the best interests of the patient, and with adequate documentation.

4. *Patient education* to provide the necessary information to the patient and family about why, how, and when medications are to be administered and their potential side effects and precautions with administration by the layperson.

Responsibility for safe administration of medications requires that the health care practitioner be familiar with every medication before administration. Knowledge of the typical and most frequently used drugs of the systems (as described in Part II of this text) is imperative. However, this is only a framework upon which to build and add other knowledge of new drugs or new effects as changes in medicine become known. Unfamiliar drugs should never be administered. Resources such as the *PDR,* the *AHFS Drug Information,* the *USP/DI,* package inserts, and pharmacists must be consulted *before* administration of a drug in order to become familiar with its desired effect, potential side effects, precautions and contraindications, and possible interactions with other drugs or with foods.

Responsibility for safe administration of medications requires *complete planning* for patient care, including prior *assessment, interventions,* and *evaluations* of the results of drug therapy. Assessment involves taking a complete history, including all medical conditions (e.g., pregnancy or illness), allergies, and all other medications in use, including over-the-counter drugs, vitamins, and herbal remedies. Assessment also involves careful observation of the patient's vital signs, posture, skin temperature and color, and facial expression before and after drug administration. Appropriate interventions require judgment in timing, discontinuing medicine if required, and taking steps to counteract adverse reactions, as well as knowing what and when to report to the physician. Evaluation and documentation of results also play a vital role for all health care providers, including the physician, in planning effective drug therapy.

The safe administration of medications necessitates training to develop skills in the delivery of medications. The goal is to maximize the effectiveness of the drug with the least discomfort to the patient. Sensitivity to the unique needs of each patient is encouraged (e.g., awareness of difficulty swallowing or impaired movement that could affect administration of medications).

Patient education is an essential part of the safe administration of medicines. If patients are to benefit from drug therapy, they must understand the importance of taking the medicine in the proper dosage, on time, and in the proper way. Information for patients should be in language they understand, with both verbal and written instructions as well as demonstrations of techniques when indicated. If the medication administration requires extra equipment or has multiple steps, a return demonstration should be required.

Administration of medication carries moral, ethical, and legal responsibilities. Some rules and regulations vary with the institution, agency, or office. When in doubt, consult those in authority—supervisors or administrators—and/or policy and procedure books. However, documentation on the patient's record is always required for all medicines given as well as for patient education. In addition, controlled substances given must also be recorded in a narcotics record as explained in Chapter 1.

# MEDICATION ERRORS

Medication errors can and do occur in all health care settings. More errors are reported from acute care settings, where the risk is greatest. However, outpatient facilities, ambulatory care sites, home health care, and long-term care facility practitioners have challenges unique to their practice as well. Patients in these settings often are older adults and likely to have several chronic conditions requiring multiple medications (see Chapter 27, "Drugs and Older Adults"). Increasing the number of medications an individual receives not only increases the risk of interactions and adverse side effects but also increases the risk of error.

Medication errors can occur in the following situations:

1. Administering a drug to the *wrong* patient
2. Administering the *wrong* drug
3. Administering a drug via the *wrong* route
4. Administering a drug at the *wrong* time
5. Administering the *wrong* dosage
6. *Wrong* documentation: improperly documenting drug administration information on a patient's medical record

Meticulous care in preparation and administration of medications reduces the chances of error. However, if a mistake is made, it is of the utmost importance to *report it* immediately to the one in charge so that corrective action can be taken for the patient's welfare. The patient's record should reflect the corrective action taken for justification in case of legal proceedings. An incident report must also be completed as a legal requirement. Failure to report errors appropriately can jeopardize the patient's welfare, as well as increase the possibility of civil suits against the health care provider and/or the risk of loss of professional license or certificate. Honesty is not only the best policy; it is the *only* policy for moral, ethical, and legal reasons.

Health care practitioners have a responsibility to provide quality care and provide for patient safety at all times. Remember, "*First, do no harm.*" This challenge includes prevention of medication errors and also reporting of medication errors so that corrective steps can be taken. As part of this goal, the U.S. Pharmacopeia (USP) has established a Medication Errors Reporting (MER) program.

In addition, the Agency for Healthcare Research and Quality (AHRQ) has federally certified the Institute for Safe Medication Practices (ISMP) as a Patient Safety Organization (PSO) to operate a national error-reporting program for both vaccine and medication errors. Health care practitioners and the public should be encouraged to report errors to ISMP since a PSO confers both privilege and confidentiality to the information reported. Error reporting by health care professionals and hospitals is necessary to develop safety alerts and quality improvement programs.

Medication reconciliation is a method used to compare the medications a patient is taking to the medications ordered by the patient's physician. This comparison is done every time there is a change in the patient's care. For example, medication reconciliation is done whenever a patient is admitted, transferred, or discharged. Medication reconciliation is done to prevent medication errors caused by omissions, duplications, errors in doses, or medication interactions (The Joint Commission, October 2012).

According to the Joint Commission, medication reconciliation consists of five steps:

1. Develop a list of current medications
2. Develop a list of medications to be prescribed
3. Compare the medications on the two lists
4. Make clinical decisions based on the comparison
5. Communicate the new list to appropriate caregivers and to the patient

# PRINCIPLES OF ADMINISTRATION

When preparing to administer medications, several basic principles should always be kept in mind:

1. *Cleanliness.* Always wash hands before handling medicines, and be sure preparation area is clean and neat.
2. *Organization.* Always be sure medications and supplies are in the appropriate area and in adequate supply. When stock drugs are used, they should be reordered immediately.
3. *Preparation area.* Should be well lighted and away from distracting influences.

Guidelines to review before administering medicines are called the Six Rights of Medication Administration (Figure 7-1):

1. Right medication
2. Right amount
3. Right time
4. Right route
5. Right patient
6. Right documentation

## Right Medication

You can confirm that you have the right medication by carefully comparing the name of the drug prescribed (on the physician's order sheet, prescription blank, medication record, or medicine card) with the label on the package, bottle,

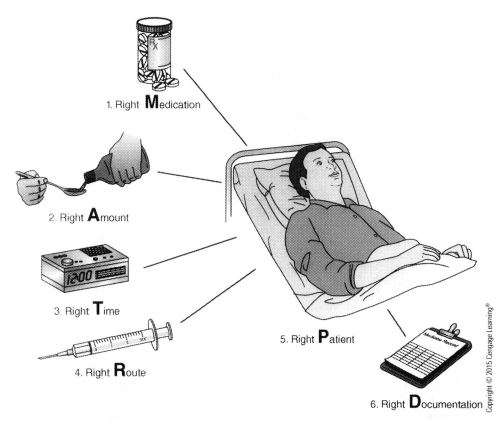

1. Right **M**edication

2. Right **A**mount

3. Right **T**ime

4. Right **R**oute

5. Right **P**atient

6. Right **D**ocumentation

**FIGURE 7-1** The Six Rights of Medication Administration.

or unit-dose packet (medications with each dose separately sealed in an individual paper, foil, plastic, or glass container). *Never* give medication when the name of the medication is obscured in any way. Some drugs have names that sound or look similar (e.g., Novolin 70/30 and Novolog Mix 70/30), and therefore it is essential to scrutinize every letter in the name when comparing the medicine ordered with the medicine on hand. Accuracy can be facilitated by placing the unit-dose packet next to the name of the drug ordered on the patient's record, while comparing the drug ordered with the drug on hand. (See Figure 8-2 in Chapter 8.)

If there is any question about the drug order because of handwriting, misspelling, inappropriateness, allergies, or interactions, you have the *right* and *responsibility to question* the physician and/or the pharmacist.

*Never* give medications that someone else has prepared. *Never* leave medications at the bedside unless specifically ordered by the physician (e.g., nitroglycerin tablets and contraceptives are frequently ordered to be left with the patient for self-administration). If the patient is unable to take a medication when you present it, the medication must be returned (in an unopened packet) to the patient's drawer in the medicine cart or medicine room. Never open the unit-dose packet until the patient is prepared to take the medicine.

## Right Amount

Administering the right amount of drug is extremely important. The drug dosage ordered must be compared *very carefully* with the dose listed on the label of the package, bottle, or unit-dose packet. Here again, accuracy can be facilitated by placing the unit-dose packet next to the written order on the patient's record while comparing the dose ordered with the dose on hand.

The three different systems of measurement (household, apothecary, and metric) were discussed in Chapter 5. It is important to consult a table of equivalents if necessary to convert from one system to another. Directions for calculation of different drug doses were presented in Chapter 6. Drug calculations are infrequent with unit-dose packaging. However, if it is necessary to compute calculations, such calculations must be checked by another trained health care practitioner, pharmacist, or physician to verify accuracy. Be especially careful when the dose is expressed in decimals or fractions. Always recheck the dose if less than ½ tablet or more than two tablets or more than 2 mL for injection is required. An unusual dosage should alert you to the possibility of error. Those who administer medications have the right, as well as the responsibility, to question any dosage that is unusual or seems inappropriate for the individual patient. Remember that drug action is influenced by the condition of the patient, metabolism, age, weight, sex, and psychological state (see Chapter 3). The health care practitioner has the responsibility of reporting the results of careful assessment and observations in order to assist the physician in prescribing the right dosage for each patient.

Directions for measurement and preparation of the right dose are described in Chapters 8 and 9. An important part of the patient education includes complete instructions about the importance of preparing and taking the right amount of medicine prescribed by the physician.

## Right Time

The time for administration of medications is an important part of the drug *dosage,* which includes the amount, frequency, and number of doses of medication to be administered. For maximum effectiveness, drugs must be given on a prescribed schedule. The physician's order specifies the number of times per day the medicine is to be administered (e.g., bid, or twice a day). Some medications need to be maintained at a specific level in the blood (*therapeutic level*) and are therefore prescribed at regular intervals around the clock (e.g., q4h or every four hours). Some medications, such as some antibiotics, are more effective on an empty stomach and are therefore prescribed *ac* (before meals). Medications that are irritating to the stomach are ordered *pc* (after meals). Drugs that cause sedation are more frequently prescribed at hour of sleep. If the physician does not prescribe a specific time for administration of a drug, the health care practitioner arranges an appropriate schedule, taking into consideration the purpose, action, and side effects of the medication. Patient education includes instruction about the right time to take specific medicines and why.

## Right Route

The route of administration is important because of its effect on degree of absorption, speed of drug action, and side effects. Many drugs can be administered in a variety of ways (see Chapter 4). The physician's order specifies the route of administration. Those administering medications have the right and responsibility to question the appropriateness of a route based on assessment and observation of the patient. Change of route may be indicated because of the patient's condition (e.g., nausea, vomiting, or difficulty swallowing). However, the route of administration may not be changed without the physician's order.

## Right Patient

The patient who is to receive the medication must be identified by use of certain techniques to reduce the chance of error. In health care facilities, the patient's wrist identification band should be checked *first,* and then the patient should be called by name or asked to state her name, *before* administering the medication. In the ambulatory care setting, the patient can be asked to give name and date of birth; this can be verified with the chart before administering medications. If the patient questions the medication or the dosage, recheck the order and the medicine before giving it.

## Right Documentation

Another essential duty is documentation of drug administration. Every medication given must be recorded on the patient's record, along with *dose, time, route,* and *location* of injections. In addition, any unusual or adverse patient reactions must be noted. If the medication is given on a PRN (as necessary) basis (e.g., for pain), notation should also be made on the patient's record of the effectiveness of the medication. The person administering the medication must also sign or initial the record after administration (the policy of each facility determines the exact procedure to be followed). The accuracy of medication documentation is a very important legal responsibility. At times, patients' records are examined in court, and the accuracy of medication documentation can be a critical factor in some legal judgments.

Documentation also includes the recording of narcotics administered on the special controlled substances record kept with the narcotics. If narcotics are destroyed because of partial dosage, cancellation, or error, two health care practitioners must sign as witnesses of the disposal of the drug (the policy about documentation of narcotics may vary with the agency).

In summary, safe and effective administration of medications involves current drug information; technical and evaluation skills; and moral, ethical, and legal responsibilities. Guidelines include the six Rights of Medication Administration. In addition, the health care practitioner has the right and responsibility to question any medication order that is confusing or illegible or that seems inappropriate and the right to refuse to administer any medication that is not in the best interests of the patient. The welfare of the patient is the primary concern in the administration of medications.

# MedWatch

The Food and Drug Administration (FDA) issued a form in 1993 to assist health care professionals in reporting serious, adverse events or product quality problems associated with medications, medical devices, or nutritional products regulated by the FDA, for example, dietary supplements or infant formulas. Even the large, well-designed clinical trials that precede FDA approval cannot uncover every problem that can come to light once a product is widely used. For example, a drug could interact with other drugs in ways that were not revealed during clinical trials. Reports by health care professionals can help ensure the safety of drugs and other products regulated by the FDA.

In response to these voluntary reports from the health care community, the FDA has issued warnings, made labeling changes, required manufacturers to do postmarketing studies, and ordered the withdrawal of certain products from the market. Such actions can prevent injuries, suffering, disabilities, congenital deformities, and even deaths.

You are not expected to establish a connection or even wait until the evidence seems overwhelming. The agency's regulations will protect your identity and the identities of your patient and your facility. With your cooperation, MedWatch can help the FDA better monitor product safety and, when necessary, take swift action to protect you and your patients. MedWatch encourages you to regard voluntary reporting as part of your professional responsibility. See Figure 7-2 for a partial MEDWATCH form and for instructions for completing and submitting this form to the FDA. In addition, you can complete a MEDWATCH online voluntary reporting form (3500) by visiting www.fda.gov/medwatch/.

U.S. Department of Health and Human Services

# MEDWATCH

**The FDA Safety Information and Adverse Event Reporting Program**

For VOLUNTARY reporting of adverse events, product problems and product use errors

Page 1 of 2

Form Approved: OMB No. 0910-0291, Expires: 6/30/2015
See PRA statement on reverse.

**FDA USE ONLY**

Triage unit sequence #

**PLEASE TYPE OR USE BLACK INK**

## A. PATIENT INFORMATION

1. Patient Identifier    2. Age at Time of Event or Date of Birth:    3. Sex ☐ Female ☐ Male    4. Weight ____ lb or ____ kg

In confidence

## B. ADVERSE EVENT, PRODUCT PROBLEM OR ERROR

Check all that apply:

1. ☐ Adverse Event   ☐ Product Problem (e.g., defects/malfunctions)
   ☐ Product Use Error   ☐ Problem with Different Manufacturer of Same Medicine

2. Outcomes Attributed to Adverse Event (Check all that apply)
   ☐ Death: ____ (mm/dd/yyyy)
   ☐ Life-threatening
   ☐ Hospitalization - initial or prolonged
   ☐ Required Intervention to Prevent Permanent Impairment/Damage (Devices)
   ☐ Disability or Permanent Damage
   ☐ Congenital Anomaly/Birth Defect
   ☐ Other Serious (Important Medical Events)

3. Date of Event (mm/dd/yyyy)    4. Date of this Report (mm/dd/yyyy)

5. Describe Event, Problem or Product Use Error

6. Relevant Tests/Laboratory Data, Including Dates

7. Other Relevant History, Including Preexisting Medical Conditions (e.g., allergies, race, pregnancy, smoking and alcohol use, liver/kidney problems, etc.)

## C. PRODUCT AVAILABILITY

Product Available for Evaluation? (Do not send product to FDA)
☐ Yes  ☐ No  ☐ Returned to Manufacturer on: ____ (mm/dd/yyyy)

## D. SUSPECT PRODUCT(S)

1. Name, Strength, Manufacturer (from product label)
#1 Name: _____ Strength: _____ Manufacturer: _____
#2 Name: _____ Strength: _____ Manufacturer: _____

2. Dose or Amount | Frequency | Route
#1
#2

3. Dates of Use (If unknown, give duration) from/to (or best estimate)
#1
#2

4. Diagnosis or Reason for Use (Indication)
#1
#2

6. Lot #   #1 #2    7. Expiration Date   #1 #2

5. Event Abated After Use Stopped or Dose Reduced?
#1 ☐ Yes ☐ No ☐ Doesn't Apply
#2 ☐ Yes ☐ No ☐ Doesn't Apply

8. Event Reappeared After Reintroduction?
#1 ☐ Yes ☐ No ☐ Doesn't Apply
#2 ☐ Yes ☐ No ☐ Doesn't Apply

9. NDC # or Unique ID

## E. SUSPECT MEDICAL DEVICE

1. Brand Name
2. Common Device Name    2b. Procode
3. Manufacturer Name, City and State
4. Model #   Catalog #   Serial #
   Lot #   Expiration Date (mm/dd/yyyy)   Unique Identifier (UDI) #
5. Operator of Device ☐ Health Professional ☐ Lay User/Patient ☐ Other:
6. If Implanted, Give Date (mm/dd/yyyy)   7. If Explanted, Give Date (mm/dd/yyyy)
8. Is this a Single-use Device that was Reprocessed and Reused on a Patient? ☐ Yes ☐ No
9. If Yes to Item No. 8, Enter Name and Address of Reprocessor

## F. OTHER (CONCOMITANT) MEDICAL PRODUCTS

Product names and therapy dates (exclude treatment of event)

## G. REPORTER (See confidentiality section on back)

1. Name and Address
   Name:
   Address:
   City:    State:    ZIP:
   Phone #    E-mail

2. Health Professional? ☐ Yes ☐ No    3. Occupation    4. Also Reported to: ☐ Manufacturer ☐ User Facility ☐ Distributor/Importer
5. If you do NOT want your identity disclosed to the manufacturer, place an "X" in this box: ☐

**FORM FDA 3500 (2/13)**   Submission of a report does not constitute an admission that medical personnel or the product caused or contributed to the event.

**FIGURE 7-2A** MedWatch form. The FDA Medical Products Reporting Program for voluntary reporting by health professionals of adverse events and product problems.

## ADVICE ABOUT VOLUNTARY REPORTING

Detailed instructions available at: http://www.fda.gov/medwatch/report/consumer/instruct.htm

**Report adverse events, product problems or product use errors with:**

- Medications *(drugs or biologics)*
- Medical devices *(including in-vitro diagnostics)*
- Combination products *(medication & medical devices)*
- Human cells, tissues, and cellular and tissue-based products
- Special nutritional products *(dietary supplements, medical foods, infant formulas)*
- Cosmetics
- Food *(including beverages and ingredients added to foods)*

**Report product problems** - quality, performance or safety concerns such as:

- Suspected counterfeit product
- Suspected contamination
- Questionable stability
- Defective components
- Poor packaging or labeling
- Therapeutic failures (product didn't work)

**Report SERIOUS adverse events. An event is serious when the patient outcome is:**

- Death
- Life-threatening
- Hospitalization - initial or prolonged
- Disability or permanent damage
- Congenital anomaly/birth defect
- Required intervention to prevent permanent impairment or damage (devices)
- Other serious (important medical events)

**Report even if:**

- You're not certain the product caused the event
- You don't have all the details

**How to report:**

- Just fill in the sections that apply to your report
- Use section D for all products except medical devices
- Attach additional pages if needed
- Use a separate form for each patient
- Report either to FDA or the manufacturer *(or both)*

**Other methods of reporting:**

- 1-800-FDA-0178 - To FAX report
- 1-800-FDA-1088 - To report by phone
- www.fda.gov/medwatch/report.htm - To report online

**If your report involves a serious adverse event with a device** and it occurred in a facility outside a doctor's office, that facility may be legally required to report to FDA and/or the manufacturer. Please notify the person in that facility who would handle such reporting.

**If your report involves a serious adverse event with a vaccine,** call 1-800-822-7967 to report.

**Confidentiality:** The patient's identity is held in strict confidence by FDA and protected to the fullest extent of the law. FDA will not disclose the reporter's identity in response to a request from the public, pursuant to the Freedom of Information Act. The reporter's identity, including the identity of a self-reporter, may be shared with the manufacturer unless requested otherwise.

-Fold Here-

-Fold Here-

---

**The information in this box applies only to requirements of the Paperwork Reduction Act of 1995**

*The burden time for this collection of information has been estimated to average 36 minutes per response, including the time to review instructions, search existing data sources, gather and maintain the data needed, and complete and review the collection of information. Send comments regarding this burden estimate or any other aspect of this collection of information, including suggestions for reducing this burden to:*

| | | |
|---|---|---|
| *Department of Health and Human Services*<br>*Food and Drug Administration*<br>*Office of Chief Information Officer*<br>*Paperwork Reduction Act (PRA) Staff*<br>*PRAStaff@fda.hhs.gov* | *Please DO NOT*<br>*RETURN this form*<br>*to the PRA Staff e-mail*<br>*to the left.* | *OMB statement:*<br>*"An agency may not conduct or sponsor, and a person is not required to respond to, a collection of information unless it displays a currently valid OMB control number."* |

**U.S. DEPARTMENT OF HEALTH AND HUMAN SERVICES**
**Food and Drug Administration**

---

FORM FDA 3500 (2/13) (Back)          Please Use Address Provided Below -- Fold in Thirds, Tape and Mail

**DEPARTMENT OF**
**HEALTH & HUMAN SERVICES**

Public Health Service
Food and Drug Administration
Rockville, MD 20857

**Official Business**
Penalty for Private Use $300

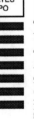

NO POSTAGE
NECESSARY
IF MAILED
IN THE
UNITED STATES
OR APO/FPO

## BUSINESS REPLY MAIL

FIRST CLASS MAIL PERMIT NO. 946 ROCKVILLE MD

POSTAGE WILL BE PAID BY FOOD AND DRUG ADMINISTRATION

*MEDWATCH*
The FDA Safety Information and Adverse Event Reporting Program
Food and Drug Administration
5600 Fishers Lane
Rockville, MD 20852-9787

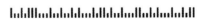

**FIGURE 7-2B** continued

# CHAPTER REVIEW QUIZ

**Complete the statements by filling in the blanks.**

1. According to the Joint Commission, medication reconciliation consists of what five steps?

2. Before administering any medication, you should have the following three pieces of information about the patient:

3. When preparing to administer medications, what three principles should be kept in mind?

4. Patient education about medication should include the following four pieces of information:

5. When administering a controlled substance, documentation is necessary in what two places?

6. Documentation of an injection given for pain should include the following five pieces of information:

7. Name the Six Rights of Drug Administration:

_____

_____

_____

_____

_____

_____

8. Medication errors must be reported immediately, and documentation includes recording the information in the following two areas:

_____

_____

| STUDYGUIDE | Online ResourcesLINK |
|---|---|
| PRACTICE | |
| Complete Chapter 7 | • PowerPoint presentations |
| | • Video |

# CHAPTER 14

## ANTINEOPLASTIC DRUGS

## Objectives

*Upon completion of this chapter, the learner should be able to*

1. Name three characteristics associated with the administration of antineoplastic drugs
2. Name and describe the major groups of antineoplastic agents
3. List the side effects common to most of the antineoplastic agents
4. Describe appropriate interventions in caring for patients receiving antineoplastic agents
5. Explain precautions in caring for those receiving radioactive isotopes
6. Describe the responsibilities of those caring for patients receiving chemotherapy
7. Explain appropriate education for the patient and family when antineoplastic agents are administered
8. List safety factors for those who care for patients receiving cytotoxic drugs
9. Define the Key Terms and Concepts

## Key Terms and Concepts

Antineoplastic
Benign
Chemotherapy
Cytotoxic
Immunosuppressive
Malignant
Palliative
Proliferating

A healthy body needs cells to reproduce and grow in an orderly, regulated manner. However, sometimes conditions are altered in the body that trigger abnormal changes in the way the cells reproduce and grow. These triggers can cause cell growth to become uncontrolled, leading to overproduction or impaired cellular development. This unregulated growth can lead to abnormal cell, tissue, and tumor development. Tumors can be classified as either benign (noncancerous) or malignant (cancerous).

Antineoplastic (against new tissue formation) refers to an agent that counteracts the development, growth, or spread of malignant cells and therefore treats various types of cancers. Cancer therapy frequently includes a combination of surgery, radiation, and chemotherapy.

Chemotherapy is a constantly growing field in which many old and new drugs and drug combinations are used for palliative effects (alleviation of symptoms) or for long-term or complete remissions in the early treatment of cancer. Antineoplastic drugs are cytotoxic (destructive to cells), especially to cells that are proliferating (reproducing rapidly). Unfortunately, the toxic effects of the antineoplastic drugs are not confined to malignant cells alone; they also affect other proliferating tissues, such as the bone marrow, gastrointestinal (GI) epithelium, skin, hair follicles, and epithelium of the gonads, resulting in numerous adverse side effects.

Significant developments continue in the use of targeted therapies that are designed to target only cancer cells, thereby sparing normal tissues. This therapy reduces host toxicity while simultaneously increasing toxicity to cancer cells and improving survival rates in patients with cancer. Many new drugs in the targeted therapy category called signal transduction inhibitors are given by the *oral route*. The first cancer *treatment* vaccine for certain men with metastatic prostate cancer was recently approved, and many others are being tested in clinical trials.

Personalized oncology medicine, utilizing pharmacogenomic biomarkers (see Chapter 3), is a developing field where based on their genetic profile, individual patients and individual cancers that respond differently to oncology medications can be identified. This is the basis for the first-line treatment of metastatic breast cancer in patients with tumors that produce excess amounts of a protein called HER2, discussed later in this chapter.

Many antineoplastic agents also possess immunosuppressive properties, because they may decrease the production of white blood cells and antibodies and reduce the inflammatory reaction. Suppression of the immune response results in increased susceptibility of the patient to infection.

Antineoplastic drugs are frequently administered in high doses on an *intermittent* schedule. Most normal tissues have a greater capacity for repair than do most malignant tissues, and therefore normal cells may recover during the drug-free period.

Chemotherapy is *individualized* and frequently modified according to the patient's response to the treatment. A *combination of several drugs* is frequently prescribed to delay the emergence of resistance, with the choice of agents based on the type of malignancy, areas involved, extent of the cancer, physical condition of the patient, and other factors. Careful planning is required to maximize the effectiveness of therapy and to minimize the side effects and discomfort for the patient. Understanding the treatment program and possible side effects is essential for all concerned: the health care practitioner, the patient, and the family. Preplanning includes provision for symptomatic relief, such as antiemetics (drugs to prevent nausea), as well as reassurance and availability of support staff to answer questions, explore feelings, and allay fears.

*The treatment of cancer is highly complex.* Only health care practitioners in oncology units, cancer treatment centers, or oncologist's offices would be expected to know the names of the numerous drugs. However, anyone who is in contact with patients on antineoplastic therapy should be aware of the frequent possible side effects and appropriate interventions for the comfort of the patient. Patient education and support are extremely important.

Antineoplastic agents can be generally classified into nine major groups: (1) antimetabolites; (2) alkylating agents; (3) mitotic inhibitors (plant alkaloids, taxanes); (4) antitumor antibiotics; (5) hormones and hormone modifiers (corticosteroids, antiestrogens, antiandrogens); (6) biological therapies (interferons, colony-stimulating factors, monoclonal antibodies); (7) targeted cancer therapies (signal transduction inhibitors); (8) vaccines; and (9) radioactive isotopes.

About one-half of all cancer patients receive some type of radiation oncology therapy sometime during the course of their treatment. Radioactive substances are placed close to or implanted in the cancerous tissues (internal radiation therapy), or an external-beam radiation is passed in three dimensions, which is made possible with computer technology.

Only one or two examples of medications are presented for each category in order to identify the side effects specific to that group. It is not necessary to remember the names of these drugs as they are only representative of the many antineoplastic agents available. However, if you work extensively with cancer patients, knowing the drug names would become important, and the National Cancer Institute website would provide you with all the latest drugs and treatments available for the various types of cancers.

# ANTIMETABOLITES

Antimetabolites work by interfering with DNA synthesis, repair, and cellular replication and are used in the treatment of various malignancies, especially those involving rapidly proliferating neoplasms (new growth). Some injectable antimetabolites include methotrexate and fluorouracil. Methotrexate is also available orally and has been used for severe, resistant cases of psoriasis, rheumatoid arthritis, and lupus. Fluorouracil is also available in a topical formulation (Efudex) to treat certain skin cancers.

Tissues that have a high rate of cellular metabolism such as neoplasms, hair follicles, buccal and GI tract lining, fetal cells, and bone marrow are most sensitive to the effects of the antimetabolites, which account for the side effects and cautions listed here.

Side effects of antimetabolites can include:

- Anorexia, nausea, vomiting, and diarrhea
- Ulceration and bleeding of the oral mucosa and GI tract
- Bone marrow suppression, including leukopenia (abnormal decrease in WBC) with infection; anemia; and thrombocytopenia (abnormal decrease in blood platelets) with hemorrhage

**NOTE**

Leucovorin (a reduced form of folic acid) is sometimes used as a "rescue agent" following methotrexate administration to reduce the side effects of methotrexate-induced hematological and GI toxicity.

⏺ Rash, itching, photosensitivity, and scaling

⏺ Alopecia (regrowth of hair may take several months)

Precautions/contraindications with antimetabolites apply to:

Renal and hepatic disorders

Pregnancy

GI ulcers

# ALKYLATING AGENTS

Alkylating agents are used in the treatment of a wide range of cancers. Some alkylating agents include cisplatin and cyclophosphamide.

These agents prevent cell growth by damaging DNA needed for reproduction. They can cause long-term damage to the bone marrow. In a few rare cases, this damage can eventually lead to acute leukemia 5 to 10 years after treatment.

Side effects of alkylating agents can include:

⏺ Nausea, vomiting, and diarrhea

⏺ Mucosal ulceration; bone marrow suppression, including leukopenia with infection; anemia; and thrombocytopenia with hemorrhage

⏺ Neurotoxicity, including headache, vertigo, and seizures

⏺ Hemorrhagic cystitis with cyclophosphamide (mesna, a chemoprotectant, can be administered prior to chemotherapy to prevent this toxicity)

Rash and alopecia

Pulmonary fibrosis

Precautions/contraindications with alkylating agents apply to:

Debilitated patients

Pregnancy

Renal disease (with cisplatin—major dose-limiting toxicity)

# MITOTIC INHIBITORS

Mitosis refers to the process of cell division and reproduction. Mitotic inhibitors are often plant alkaloids and other compounds derived from natural products that block mitosis. They are used to treat many different types of cancer. These agents are also known for their potential to cause peripheral nerve damage and myelosuppression, which can be dose-limiting side effects.

# Plant Alkaloids

Plant alkaloids, for example vinblastine or vincristine, which are derived from the periwinkle plant, are used in combination with other chemotherapeutic agents in the treatment of various malignancies. Vinorelbine (Navelbine), a semisynthetic agent derived from vinblastine, has been recommended as a treatment of choice for lung cancer in older patients.

Side effects of plant alkaloids can include:

- Neurotoxicity, including numbness; tingling; ataxia; foot drop; pain in the jaw, head, or extremities; and visual disturbances (less common with vinblastine and vinorelbine)
- Severe constipation or diarrhea, nausea, and vomiting
- Oral or GI ulceration
- Rash, phototoxicity (increased reaction to sunlight), and alopecia

  Leukopenia with vinblastine (hematological effects less common with vincristine)

  Necrosis of tissue if intravenous drug solution infiltrates into tissues (for IV cannula placement, avoid areas of previous irradiation and extremities with poor venous circulation).

Precautions/contraindications with plant alkaloids apply to:

Pregnancy

Hepatic dysfunction

Infection

Geriatric patients

**NOTE**

Intrathecal administration (into the spinal canal) of these agents is fatal. This route must not be used. Syringes containing these agents should be labeled, "Warning—For IV use only, fatal if given intrathecally."

# Taxanes

Paclitaxel, another plant alkaloid, was originally extracted from the bark of the Western (Pacific) yew. It is structurally different from other available antineoplastic agents. It is used as a second-line or subsequent therapy in patients with metastatic breast or ovarian carcinoma refractory to conventional chemotherapy.

Adverse side effects of paclitaxel are frequent and include:

- Bone marrow suppression: neutropenia, leukopenia, thrombocytopenia, and anemia
- Hypersensitivity reactions—can be severe, with flushing, rash, dyspnea, chest pain, hypotension, and bradycardia
- Peripheral neuropathy (occurs in up to 30% of patients)
- Nausea, vomiting, diarrhea, and mucositis (inflammation of the mucous membranes)
- Alopecia

  Necrosis of tissue if intravenous drug solution infiltrates into tissues

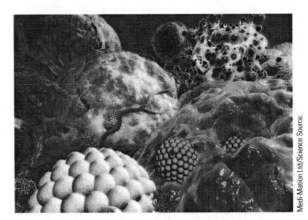

**FIGURE 14-1** Illustration of nanoparticles (blue) containing cytotoxic drugs and targeting the tumor cells (purple). The orange cells represent dead and dying tumor cells.

Precautions/contraindications with paclitaxel apply to:

Pregnancy

Hepatic dysfunction

Infection

Cardiac disease

Due to its severe adverse reactions, paclitaxel is administered only by IV under constant supervision of an oncologist, with frequent monitoring of vital signs and facilities available for emergency interventions if required.

Just to show the "Star Trek" quality of research in cancer medications, NAB-paclitaxel (Abraxane) is the first approved albumin nanoparticle drug. Paclitaxel is mixed with albumin nanoparticles (one billionth of a meter in size), which act as biological delivery agents to transport the drug to the needed site of action. See Figure 14-1 for a rendering of how nanoparticles work.

# ANTITUMOR ANTIBIOTICS

Antitumor antibiotics are used to treat a wide variety of malignancies. Doxorubicin (Adriamycin) is considered the most active chemotherapy agent and is a critical component in the treatment protocols of breast, lung, gastric, and ovarian cancers and lymphoma, but it can permanently damage the heart if given in high doses. Daunorubicin (Cerubidine), which is structurally related to doxorubicin, is primarily used for acute leukemias due to its lower incidence of cardiotoxicity. Other antitumor antibiotics include bleomycin and mitomycin. They are frequently used in combination with other drugs.

> **NOTE**
>
> Side effects vary depending on specific medications. Always check side effects for each drug in this classification.

Side effects of antitumor antibiotics can include:

- Anorexia, nausea, vomiting, and diarrhea
- Bone marrow suppression (the acute dose-limiting toxicity with doxorubicin and daunorubicin)

- Cardiotoxicity, including arrhythmias; congestive heart failure and cardiomyopathy (cumulative dosing with most medications except bleomycin)
- Pneumonitis and dyspnea; pulmonary fibrosis with bleomycin
- Ulceration of the mouth or colon
- Alopecia, rash, and scaling

  Tissue necrosis if intravenous solution infiltrates (with most meds)

Precautions/contraindications with antitumor antibiotics apply to:

Pregnancy

Liver disorders

Cardiac disease

# HORMONES AND HORMONE MODIFIERS

Hormones used in the treatment of cancer include the corticosteroids. Hormone modifiers include the antiestrogen and the antiandrogen agents.

## Corticosteroids

*Corticosteroids,* such as prednisone, are used primarily for their suppressant effect on lymphocytes in leukemias and lymphomas. They are also frequently used in combination with other chemotherapeutic agents in the treatment of some types of cancer and before chemotherapy to help prevent severe allergic reactions. In addition, large doses of dexamethasone have been found to be effective in the prevention and treatment of nausea and vomiting associated with many antineoplastic agents, when administered before or during chemotherapy. Dexamethasone is also used to treat cerebral edema associated with brain tumors.

Side effects with prolonged use of corticosteroids (see Chapter 23 for a more detailed listing) include:

- Fluid retention, edema

  Cushingoid features (moon face)
- Nausea/vomiting, gastritis, and GI bleeding
- Osteoporosis with fractures

## Antiestrogens

A *nonsteroidal* agent belonging to a class of drugs called selective estrogen-receptor modifiers (SERMs), tamoxifen, binds to estrogen receptors in various tissues. It can be used as a primary hormonal therapy both for metastatic estrogen receptor–positive breast cancer in both men and postmenopausal women and also for palliative treatment. Tamoxifen also stimulates estrogen receptors in bones and may help prevent osteoporosis.

Serious adverse side effects are rare and usually dose related. Nausea, vomiting, hot flashes, and night sweats can occur in up to 66% of cases but usually do not require discontinuation of the medication. Antidepressants may be prescribed to alleviate tamoxifen-associated hot flashes. Some antidepressants may reduce the potency of tamoxifen.

Anastrozole (Arimidex) and letrozole (Femara), which inhibit the final step in estrogen production, offer alternatives to tamoxifen in postmenopausal women with breast cancer. They can also cause nausea, vomiting, and hot flashes similar to tamoxifen but are more likely than tamoxifen to cause osteoporosis.

## Antiandrogens

*Antiandrogen* drugs include leuprolide acetate, which suppresses testosterone production in the testes and is usually administered IM (Lupron Depot) or SC (Eligard) on monthly regimens (every one, three, four, or six depending on the dosage) for prostate cancer. They are also used as hormonal therapy in the treatment of endometriosis. See Chapter 24 for more details.

Bicalutamide (Casodex) is an oral nonsteroidal antiandrogen, which interferes with the binding of testosterone to androgen receptors in the prostate and is used simultaneously with leuprolide in the treatment of metastatic prostate cancer.

Side effects of antiandrogens can include:

- Impotence
- Hot flashes, generalized pain, infection, constipation, and nausea

Patients should be advised that the drug be continued even when signs or symptoms of the disease improve.

*Sex hormones,* including the estrogens, progestins, and androgens, are also used as antineoplastic agents in the treatment of malignancies involving the reproductive system (e.g., cancer of the breast, uterus, or prostate). These hormones are discussed in Chapter 24.

## BIOLOGICAL THERAPIES

Biological therapy (also called immunotherapy, biotherapy, or biological response modifier therapy) is designed to repair, stimulate, or enhance cancer patients' natural immune systems to more effectively recognize and attack cancer cells. Some therapies are used to lessen the side effects caused by certain cancer treatments. There are different types of immunotherapy: The *active* or *direct* type (such as interferons) stimulates the body's own immune system to fight the disease. The *passive* or *indirect* type (such as monoclonal antibodies) uses immune system components created outside the body.

## Interferons

Interferon alfa (Intron A), which is the type most widely used in cancer treatments, is a complex combination of many proteins that boost immune system response. Its antiviral action is described in Chapter 17. Interferons are used in the treatment of certain leukemias, melanoma, Kaposi's sarcoma, and non-Hodgkin's lymphoma. Interferons are also used to treat hepatitis B and C, multiple sclerosis, and other conditions.

Adverse side effects of interferons, sometimes severe, are experienced by almost all patients receiving interferon, varying with the dosage and condition. Most common side effects include:

- Flulike syndrome—fever, fatigue, chills, headache, muscle aches, and pains
- GI symptoms—anorexia, nausea, vomiting, diarrhea, and dry mouth
- Nervous system effects—sleep disturbances, depression, and neuropathy
- Hematological effects—especially leukopenia and anemia
  Dyspnea, cough, nasal congestion, and pneumonia
  Alopecia—transient

# COLONY-STIMULATING FACTORS

Colony-stimulating factors (CSFs) such as erythropoietin (Epogen, Procrit) usually do not directly affect tumor cells. They encourage bone marrow stem cells to divide and develop into red and white blood cells and platelets. Since anticancer drugs can damage the body's ability to make these cells, patients have an increased risk of developing infections, becoming anemic, and bleeding more easily. By using CSFs to stimulate blood cell production, oncologists can increase the doses of antineoplastics without increasing the risk of infection or the need for transfusions.

Refer to Chapter 25 for other uses of CSFs and their side effects.

# MONOCLONAL ANTIBODIES

Monoclonal antibodies (MABs) are *exogenous* (*outside of body*) antibodies genetically engineered in the laboratory. MABs are designed to target only cancer cells, thereby sparing normal tissues (i.e., not *directly* cytotoxic). This reduces host toxicity while simultaneously increasing toxicity to cancer cells. One specific type of MAB is indicated where tumors have rich blood supplies, which can facilitate their growth and spread. Angiogenesis inhibitors (AIs) prevent the formation of new blood vessels that tumors need to grow and invade nearby tissue. Bevacizumab (Avastin), in combination with other agents, is indicated for the first-line treatment of patients with metastatic carcinoma of the highly vascularized colon, kidney, or lung. AIs may only stop or slow the growth of a cancer, not completely eradicate it.

Another MAB, trastuzumab (Herceptin), combined with paclitaxel, is indicated for first-line treatment of metastatic breast cancer in patients with tumors that produce excess amounts of a protein called HER2. *All MABs are administered intravenously.*

Side effects of MABs are common, especially with the first infusion, and can include:

- Fever and chills, headache, and dizziness
- Nausea and vomiting

  Itching, rash, and generalized pain

These reactions should occur less frequently with subsequent infusions.

Severe reactions can be minimized by *premedicating* with acetaminophen (Tylenol), diphenhydramine (Benadryl), and/or meperidine (Demerol). AIs (Avastin) may have side effects that are different from other MABs. Signs of severe reaction can include:

- Angioedema, hypotension, dyspnea, and bronchospasm (may be necessary to stop infusion)
- Hypersensitivity reactions (including anaphylaxis)
- Cardiac arrhythmias, angina, heart failure, cardiomyopathy; hypertensive crisis (with Avastin)

  Acute renal failure (not with Herceptin)
- Hematological toxicity (i.e., reduced white blood cells [WBCs]); complete blood count (CBC) and platelet count should be monitored frequently
- GI perforation, GI bleed; impaired wound healing (all with Avastin)

# TARGETED THERAPIES

Targeted cancer therapies are drugs or other substances that block the growth and spread of cancer by interfering with specific molecules involved in tumor growth and progression. By focusing on molecular and cellular changes that are specific to cancer, targeted cancer therapies may be more effective than other types of treatment, including chemotherapy and radiotherapy, and are less harmful to normal cells.

## Signal Transduction Inhibitors

One of the newer and largest grouping of targeted therapy drugs are called the signal transduction inhibitors (STIs), which block specific enzymes and growth factor receptors that signal cancer cell proliferation. Imatinib (Gleevec) is one of the first clinically useful agents in this class and is approved for the treatment of chronic myelogenous leukemia and some rare types of cancers. The majority of STIs are given by the *oral* route. Side effects vary greatly depending on the indication, agent, and combination therapy used.

# VACCINES

Vaccines are medicines that boost the immune system's natural ability to protect the body against "foreign invaders," mainly infectious agents that may cause disease. There are two broad types of cancer vaccines:

 * *Preventive (or prophylactic),* which are intended to prevent cancer from developing in healthy people
 * *Treatment (or therapeutic),* which are intended to treat an existing cancer by strengthening the body's natural defenses against the cancer.

The FDA has approved two vaccines, Gardasil and Cervarix, that *protect* against infection by the two types of human papilloma virus (HPV) that cause approximately 70 percent of all cases of cervical cancer worldwide. Neither vaccine is indicated for the *treatment* of HPV infection and will not protect against all HPV types not contained within the vaccine. Therefore, recipients of the vaccine should continue to undergo routine cervical and anal cancer screenings.

Patients who have latex hypersensitivity may be inappropriate candidates for the Cervarix prefilled syringe, as the tip cap and the rubber plunger of the needleless prefilled syringes contain dry, natural latex rubber.

The first cancer *treatment* vaccine, sipuleucel-T (Provenge), is approved for use in some men with metastatic prostate cancer. Sipuleucel-T is made from a patient's white blood cells to stimulate the patient's immune system against the cancer and is manufactured for each patient individually.

See Chapter 17 for a discussion of traditional vaccines.

# RADIOACTIVE ISOTOPES

Radioactive isotopes are also used in the treatment of certain types of cancer. Sometimes the radioactive material is injected into the affected site (e.g., radiogold, injected into the pleural or peritoneal cavity to treat the abnormal accumulation of fluid called ascites caused by the cancer). Radioactive sodium iodide is administered PO to treat thyroid cancer (thyroid cells naturally take up radioactive iodine). Radioactive material is sometimes implanted in the body in the form of capsules, needles, or seeds.

The newest targeted therapy provides the added benefit of radiation.

Radioimmunotherapy consists of MABs that have radioisotopes attached to them so that whatever the targeted antibody binds to can also be irradiated. Tositumomab (Bexxar) with iodine 131 is indicated for patients with refractory non-Hodgkin's lymphoma. The primary side effect after radioimmunotherapy is a decreased blood count occurring four to six weeks after treatment. The counts remain low for two to three weeks and then returns to normal. The distinct advantage of radioimmunotherapy is that it is usually given one time.

Health care practitioners caring for patients receiving radioactive isotopes must observe special precautions to prevent unnecessary radiation exposure. Gowns and gloves should be worn when handling patient excreta such as feces, urine, and body secretions. Other isolation procedures, such as handling of linens, will be outlined in the facility's procedure manual. This protocol should be followed with great care by all those who come in contact with patients receiving radioactive materials, for the protection of patients as well as the health care practitioner.

# CAUTIONS AND RESPONSIBILITIES FOR ANTINEOPLASTIC DRUGS

Health care practitioners involved in the administration of antineoplastic agents, as well as those who care for these patients, have a number of very important responsibilities.

1.  All medications should be given on time and exactly as prescribed to keep the patient as comfortable as possible and maximize the efficacy and safety of the medication. Check package inserts on all new drugs.

2.  Intravenous sites must be checked with great care because some antineoplastic agents (especially antitumor antibiotics and vinca alkaloids) can cause extreme tissue damage and necrosis if infiltration into surrounding tissues occurs. (Gloves should be worn when handling IVs with antineoplastic agents.) Facilities may have a kit available containing supplies and medications needed to treat extravasation.

3.  Intravenous fluids containing antineoplastic agents should not be allowed to get on the skin or into the eyes of the patient or the one administering the medication. Flush skin or eyes copiously if spills occur.

4.  Antiemetics should be immediately available and administered as prescribed to minimize nausea and vomiting. Ondansetron (Zofran) and dolasetron (Anzemet) are examples of antiemetics used for this purpose (see Chapter 16).

5.  Careful and frequent oral hygiene is essential to minimize discomfort and ulceration.

6.  Soft foods and cool liquids should be available to the patient as required.

7.  Accurate intake and output is important for the adequate assessment of hydration.

8.  Careful observation and reporting of symptoms and side effects is an essential part of chemotherapy.

9.  Aseptic technique is necessary to minimize the chance of infection in patients with reduced resistance to infection.

10. Careful assessment of vital signs is important to identify the signs of infection, cardiac irregularities, and dyspnea.

11. The health care practitioner and family must be informed about all aspects of chemotherapy and answer the patient's questions honestly. Awareness of verbal and nonverbal communication that gives clues to the patient's needs is absolutely necessary.

12. Careful attention to detail, astute observations, appropriate interventions, and compassion are an integral part of care when the patient is receiving chemotherapy.

13. The health care practitioner should reassure the patient that someone will be available to help at all times and should identify all resources available for both the patient and his or her family.

# PATIENT EDUCATION

Patients being treated with antineoplastic drugs and their families should be instructed regarding:

Side effects to expect, how long they can be expected to continue, and that they are frequently temporary

Comfort measures for coping with unpleasant side effects (e.g., antiemetics and antidiarrheal agents as prescribed)

Appropriate diet with foods that are more palatable and more likely to be tolerated (e.g., soft foods, bland foods, a variety of liquids, and especially cold foods in frequent, small quantities)

Careful aseptic technique to decrease the chance of infections and reporting any signs of infection (e.g., fever)

Careful oral hygiene with swabs to prevent further trauma to ulcerated mucosa

Observation for bleeding in stools, urine, and gums and for bruises, and reporting this to medical personnel

Reporting any persistent or unusual side effects, such as dizziness, severe headache, numbness, tingling, difficulty walking, or visual disturbances

Available community resources to assist and support the patient (e.g., Cancer Society, Hospice, or Home Health Services) as required and recommended by the physician

How to obtain information and answers to questions regarding treatment

The right of patients to terminate therapy if they wish

See Table 14-1 for a summary of antineoplastic agents' side effects.

## Cytotoxic Drug Dangers to Health Care Personnel

Most cytotoxic drugs are toxic substances known to be carcinogenic, mutagenic, or teratogenic. Anyone who prepares, administers, or cares for patients receiving cytotoxic drugs should be aware of the dangers involved. The American Society of Health-System Pharmacists (ASHP) has published a *Technical Assistance Bulletin (TAB)* that provides detailed advice on recommended policies, procedures, and equipment for the safe handling of cytotoxic drugs (see AHFS Drug Information). It is essential that policies and procedures be followed exactly as outlined on the labels provided by the drug company. Guidelines of the individual health care agency must also be followed to the letter for the safety of all concerned.

**TABLE 14-1** Side Effects of Antineoplastic Agents

| POSSIBLE SIDE EFFECTS | DRUG CATEGORIES | | | | | | | |
|---|---|---|---|---|---|---|---|---|
| | ANTIMETABOLITES | ALKYLATING AGENTS | MITOTIC INHIBITORS (PLANT ALKALOIDS) | ANTITUMOR ANTIBIOTICS | HORMONE AND HORMONE MODIFIERS | INTERFERONS | MONOCLONAL ANTIBODIES (MABs) | SIGNAL TRANSDUCTION INHIBITORS |
| GI effects: nausea, vomiting, diarrhea | X | X | X | X | X | X | X | X |
| Alopecia | X | X | X | X | | X | | |
| Suppressed bone marrow[a] | X | X | X | X | | X (especially leukopenia) | X | |
| Ulcerated mucosa | X | X | X | X | | | X | |
| Photosensitivity | X | | X | | | | | |
| Neurotoxicity | X | X | X | | | X | | |
| Hypersensitivity | | | X | | | | X | X |
| Cardiotoxicity | | | | X | | | X | X |
| Respiratory dysfunction | X | X | | X | | X | X | X |
| Hot flashes | | | | | X | | | |
| Impotence | | | | | X | | | |
| Flu-like syndrome | | | | | | X | X | X |
| Renal toxicity | | X | | | | | | X |

[a]Includes leukopenia (low WBC count) and prone to infections, anemias, thrombocytopenia, and hemorrhage.

The danger to health care personnel from handling a hazardous drug stems from a combination of its inherent toxicity and the extent to which practitioners are exposed in the course of carrying out their duties. This exposure may be from inadvertent ingestion of the drug on foodstuffs, inhalation of drug dust or droplets, or direct skin contact.

Recommended safe handling methods include four broad goals:

1. Protect and secure packages of hazardous drugs. Store them separately from nonhazardous drugs.

2. Inform and educate all involved personnel about hazardous drugs and train them in safe handling procedures.

3. Do not let the drugs escape from containers when they are manipulated (i.e., dissolved, transferred, administered, or discarded).

4. Eliminate the possibility of inadvertent ingestion or inhalation and direct skin or eye contact with the drugs.

Specific recommendations for cytotoxic drugs include:

1. When preparing these drugs, wear gloves, long-sleeved gowns, splash goggles, and disposable respirator masks.

2. For administration, wear long-sleeved gowns and gloves. Syringes and IV sets with Luer-Lock fittings should be used, and care should be taken that all fittings are secure.

3. Dispose of syringes, IV tubing and bags, gauze, or any other contaminated material such as linens in a leak proof, puncture-resistant container that is labeled "HAZARD."

4. Wear gloves and gown when handling excreta from patients receiving cytotoxic drugs.

5. Those who are pregnant, breast-feeding, or actively trying to conceive a child should not care for patients receiving cytotoxic drugs.

For more detailed instructions, see *ASHP Technical Assistance Bulletin on Handling Cytotoxic and Hazardous Drugs,* which is reproduced in the AHFS Drug Information book and updated based on information from Occupational Safety and Health Administration (OSHA), National Institutes of Health (NIH), National Study Commission on Cytotoxic Exposure, and the American Medical Association (AMA) Council on Scientific Affairs.

Antineoplastic therapy is complex and changes frequently with ongoing research. Therefore, you are not expected to remember the names of all of the antineoplastic agents. However, you need to know the *common side effects, interventions, cautions, and appropriate patient education.*

# CASE STUDY A

## ANTINEOPLASTIC DRUGS

The oncology infusion clinic's first patient of the day is Herman Johnson, a 72-year-old male with a new diagnosis of metastatic colon cancer. The oncologist has ordered a medication from a category of drugs as a first-line treatment that will *not* eradicate the cancer but *will* stop or slow the growth of cancer.

1. This category of drug is called a(n):
   a. Colony stimulating factor
   b. Vaccine
   c. Angiogenesis inhibitor
   d. Signal transduction inhibitor

2. Upon receiving his first dose, the nurse informs Mr. Johnson that he can expect which symptom(s)?
   a. Fever and chills
   b. Hot flashes
   c. Decreased platelet count
   d. Blood in his stools

3. Prior to a first dose, the nurse will administer which medication to minimize a potentially severe reaction?
   a. Morphine sulfate
   b. Motrin
   c. Mylanta
   d. Benadryl

4. During an infusion of Avastin, the nurse will be watching out for which possible side effect that may necessitate stopping the infusion?
   a. Nausea
   b. Bronchospasm
   c. Metallic taste in the mouth
   d. Headache

5. In the next several weeks, Mr. Johnson will be monitored for which side effect?
   a. Hypotension
   b. Low WBCs
   c. Constipation
   d. Excessive bruising

# CASE STUDY B

## ANTINEOPLASTIC DRUGS

During 39-year-old Geneva Moyet's annual physical, a physician palpates a swollen thyroid gland. A CT scan and biopsy determines that she has thyroid cancer. The physician refers her to an oncologist, who indicates that she should be treated with radioactive sodium iodide, a radioisotope.

1. With which route will this specific radioisotope be administered?
   a. Intramuscular injection
   b. Seed placement
   c. Orally
   d. Intravenously

2. What is a distinct advantage of radioimmunotherapy?
   a. It is usually given one time.
   b. It has no side effects.
   c. It is given once a month.
   d. No extra precautions need to be taken post-treatment.

3. Which of the following is the primary side effect of radioimmunotherapy?
   a. Diarrhea
   b. Nausea
   c. Fever
   d. Decreased blood count

4. Which should the nurse wear when handling patient excreta after radioimmunotherapy?
   a. Gloves only
   b. Gown and gloves
   c. Cap, gown, and gloves
   d. Cap, gown, gloves, and booties

5. Suppose that Geneva develops a low blood count. What category of drug would be given to her that would stimulate the bone marrow production of red and white blood cells as well as platelets?
   a. Colony-stimulating factor
   b. Hormone modifiers
   c. Biological therapy (interferons)
   d. Antitumor antibiotics

# CHAPTER REVIEW QUIZ

**Match the term with the definition:**

1. _____ Palliative
2. _____ Cytotoxic
3. _____ Antineoplastic
4. _____ Monoclonal antibodies
5. _____ Proliferating
6. _____ Exogenous antibodies
7. _____ Refractory
8. _____ Immunosuppressive
9. _____ Endogenous antibodies
10. _____ Clone

a. Target only cancer cells
b. Unresponsive to treatment
c. Within the cell
d. Produce a copy
e. Decreases antibody production
f. Alleviation of symptoms
g. Engineered in a laboratory
h. Reproducing rapidly
i. Destructive to cells
j. Counteracts malignant cell growth

## Multiple Choice

11. Alkylating agents such as cisplatin and cyclophosphamide work by which method of action?

   a. They prevent growth by damaging DNA needed for reproduction.
   b. They assist in bone marrow depression.
   c. They block cell mitosis.
   d. They bind to estrogen receptors.

12. A tumor that is classified as benign is:

   a. Destructive to other cells
   b. Noncancerous
   c. Cancerous
   d. Resistant to radiation

13. A common side effect of an antimetabolite is:

   a. Numbness and tingling
   b. Phototoxicity
   c. Nausea and vomiting
   d. Visual disturbances

14. Which drug is used to treat cerebral edema associated with brain tumors?

   a. Leucovorin
   b. Anastrozole
   c. Letrozole
   d. Dexamethasone

15. Which antitumor antibiotic is known to be cardiotoxic and can permanently damage the heart if given in high doses?

   a. Mitomycin
   b. Daunorubicin
   c. Adriamycin
   d. Bleomycin

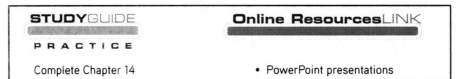

STUDYGUIDE

PRACTICE

Complete Chapter 14

Online ResourcesLINK

• PowerPoint presentations

# CHAPTER 16
## GASTROINTESTINAL DRUGS

## Objectives

*Upon completion of this chapter, the learner should be able to*

1. Describe uses, side effects, precautions and contraindications, and interactions of antacids, antiulcer and agents for GERD, agents for IBS, antidiarrheal agents, antiflatulents, cathartics and laxatives, and antiemetics

2. Compare and contrast the seven types of laxatives according to use, side effects, precautions and contraindications, and interactions

3. Identify examples of drugs from each of the eight categories of gastrointestinal drugs

4. Explain important patient education for each category of gastrointestinal drugs

5. Differentiate causes and treatment of *H. pylori* and *C. difficile* infections

6. Define the Key Terms and Concepts

## Key Terms and Concepts

Antacids

Antidiarrheal

Antiemetics

Antiflatulents

GI Antispasmodic

Antiulcer

Chemotherapy-induced nausea and vomiting (CINV)

Gastroesophageal reflux disease (GERD)

Histamine₂ blockers

Inflammatory bowel disease (IBD)

Laxatives

Postoperative nausea and vomiting (PONV)

Probiotics

Proton pump inhibitor (PPI)

According to the National Institutes of Health, 60 to 70 million people suffer from digestive diseases. Gastrointestinal drugs covered in this chapter can be divided into the following eight categories based on their mechanism of action:

Antacids

Drugs for treatment of ulcers and gastroesophageal reflux disease (GERD)

GI Antispasmodics

Agents for inflammatory bowel disease

Antidiarrheal agents

Antiflatulents

Laxatives and cathartics

Antiemetics

# ANTACIDS

*Pyrosis,* commonly known as heartburn, and *dyspepsia* (acid indigestion) are experienced by up to 40% of the population in the United States at least once a month. Antacids act by partially neutralizing gastric hydrochloric acid and are widely available in many over-the-counter (OTC) preparations for the relief of indigestion, heartburn, and sour stomach. Other antiulcer agents are discussed later in this chapter. Antacids are also used at times as supplemental agents in the management of esophageal reflux.

Antacid products may contain aluminum, calcium carbonate, or magnesium, either individually or in combination. Most antacids also contain sodium. Sodium bicarbonate alone is not recommended because of flatulence, metabolic alkalosis, and electrolyte imbalance with prolonged use. Calcium carbonate, for example Tums, is rapid acting and possesses good neutralizing capacity but may cause constipation and kidney stones if overused.

The choice of a specific antacid preparation depends on palatability, cost, adverse effects, acid-neutralizing capacity, sodium content, and the patient's renal and cardiovascular function. Generally, antacids have a short duration of action, requiring frequent administration. Magnesium and/or aluminum antacids are the most commonly used. Magnesium can cause diarrhea, and aluminum causes constipation. Therefore, combinations, for example Maalox, Gelusil, and Mylanta, are frequently used to control the frequency and consistency of bowel movements.

Side effects with the frequent use of antacids may include:

- Constipation (with aluminum or calcium carbonate antacids)
- Diarrhea (with magnesium antacids)
- Electrolyte imbalance
- Urinary calculi (stone formation) and renal complications
- Osteoporosis (with aluminum antacids)
- Belching and flatulence (with calcium carbonate and sodium bicarbonate)

Precautions or contraindications with antacids apply to:

Heart failure

Chronic kidney disease or history of renal calculi

Cirrhosis of the liver or edema

Dehydration or electrolyte imbalance

Antacids may either increase or decrease the absorption of other medications. For many medications, this interaction does not result in patient harm. However, because they may decrease the effectiveness of the drug, antacids should not be taken within 2h of administering the following medications:

Anti-infectives, especially tetracyclines, quinolones, and isoniazid

Digoxin, indomethacin, and iron

Salicylates and thyroid hormones

Bisphosphonates (i.e., Actonel, Fosamax)

Antacids with the following drugs may increase action and precipitate side effects:

Diazepam, which increases sedation

Amphetamines and quinidine, which increase cardiac irregularities

Enteric-coated drugs may be released prematurely in the stomach (separate doses from antacids by 2h).

## PATIENT EDUCATION

Patients using antacids should be instructed regarding:

Avoiding prolonged use (no longer than two weeks) of OTC antacids without medical supervision because of the danger of masking symptoms of gastrointestinal (GI) bleeding or GI malignancy and causing the stomach to increase excess acid

Avoiding the use of antacids at the same time as any other medication because of many interactions (check with a pharmacist or physician concerning clinically important interactions)

Avoiding the use of antacids entirely or use with caution if the patient has cardiac, renal, or liver disease or fluid retention

Patients taking medicines for the management of esophageal reflux should also be instructed regarding avoidance of constrictive clothing, treatment of obesity (if appropriate), reducing meal size, avoiding lying down after meals, restriction of alcohol use, elimination of smoking, and elevating the head of the bed during sleep.

# AGENTS FOR TREATMENT OF ULCERS AND GASTROESOPHAGEAL REFLUX DISEASE

## H$_2$-Blockers

The histamine receptors found in the stomach are called H$_2$-receptors. H$_2$-receptor antagonists *reduce gastric acid secretion* by acting as histamine$_2$ blockers. They also reduce the amount of gastric acid released in response to stimuli such as food and caffeine. The drugs in this category, cimetidine, famotidine (Pepcid), and ranitidine (Zantac), are used *short term* for the relief of "acid indigestion and heartburn," gastroesophageal reflux disease (GERD), esophagitis, and prevention of duodenal ulcer recurrence.

Side effects of H$_2$-blockers, usually transient and dose related, can include:

Diarrhea, dizziness, rash, and headache

Mild gynecomastia with cimetidine occurs infrequently and is reversible

Mental confusion (especially in older or debilitated adults; less with Pepcid)

Precautions or contraindications with H$_2$-blockers apply to:

Renal disease (may need to reduce dose and/or frequency)

Pregnancy

Lactation

Interactions with cimetidine may occur with increased blood concentrations of:

Warfarin (Coumadin) (also with high doses of Zantac)

Phenytoin

Beta-blockers

Benzodiazepines

Lidocaine

Theophylline (also with high doses of Zantac)

Tricyclic antidepressants

Proton pump inhibitors may interfere with the effectiveness of H$_2$-blockers; when given together the H$_2$-blocker is usually given at bedtime

**NOTE**

There is less likelihood for drug interactions with Pepcid.

All the H$_2$-blockers are available OTC for up to two weeks of self-treatment; beyond that time frame a physician should be consulted.

## Proton Pump Inhibitors

GERD is caused by the excessive reflux of acidic gastric contents into the esophagus, resulting in irritation or injury to the esophageal mucosa characterized by heartburn and acid regurgitation. Serious complications include esophageal stricture, pulmonary aspiration, and esophageal cancer.

Omeprazole (Prilosec) is a gastric antisecretory agent (proton pump inhibitor or PPI), unrelated to the H$_2$-receptor antagonists. It is used for the *short-term* (four to eight weeks) symptomatic relief of GERD, for the *short-term* treatment of *confirmed* gastric and duodenal ulcers, and for erosive esophagitis and "heartburn." PPIs may be used *long-term* for severe GERD, preventing NSAID-induced ulcers, and hypersecretory conditions. Other drugs in this category include lansoprazole (Prevacid), rabeprazole (Aciphex), pantoprazole (Protonix), and esomeprazole (Nexium).

Side effects of PPIs can include:

- Diarrhea, constipation, nausea, vomiting, and abdominal pain
- Increased risk for pneumonia or intestinal (*Clostridium difficile*) infection

  Long-term use on a regular basis of agents that reduce gastric acid can possibly result in vitamin B$_{12}$ deficiency and low magnesium levels in the blood, especially in older adults.

  In patients older than 50 years, long-term PPI therapy (at least one year), particularly at high doses, is also associated with an increased risk of hip, wrist, or spine fractures. A potential mechanism for this is PPIs' interference with calcium absorption.

Interactions of PPIs may occur with:

Clopidogrel (Plavix) (a platelet inhibitor; see Chapter 25)

$H_2$-blockers (decrease PPI effectiveness)

Sucralfate (delays absorption of most PPIs)

Benzodiazepines, phenytoin, and warfarin (increased serum levels)

Ampicillin, ketoconazole, iron salts, vitamin $B_{12}$, bisphosphonates (results in poor bioavailability)

Food—Nexium, Prevacid, and Prilosec should be given on an empty stomach; Aciphex and Protonix can be given without regard to meals.

# GASTRIC MUCOSAL AGENTS

## Misoprostol (Cytotec)

Misoprostol (Cytotec), a synthetic form of prostaglandin $E_1$, inhibits gastric acid secretion and protects the mucosa from the irritant effect of certain drugs, for example nonsteroidal anti-inflammatory drugs (NSAIDs—see Chapter 21), especially in those at risk, for example debilitated patients or older adults or those with a history of gastric ulcers. It is not FDA approved for the treatment of gastric or duodenal ulcers that are *unrelated* to NSAID use.

Side effects of Cytotec can include:

Diarrhea, nausea, and abdominal pain (occurs early in the treatment and is usually self-limiting; take with food to minimize effects)

Menstrual irregularities (begin therapy on the second or third day of the next normal menstrual period)

Spontaneous abortion, possibly incomplete, with potentially dangerous uterine bleeding or maternal or fetal death

Precautions or contraindications for Cytotec include:

Women of childbearing age (unless the woman is capable of using effective contraceptives)

Pregnant women

Children under age 12

Interactions with antacids decrease the rate of absorption. Therefore, it is recommended that antacids should be given at least 2h away and should not be of a magnesium type (which exacerbates diarrhea).

## Sucralfate (Carafate)

Sucralfate (Carafate), an inhibitor of pepsin, is another antiulcer agent that acts in a different way. Sucralfate is *administered on an empty stomach* and then reacts with hydrochloric acid in the stomach to form a paste that adheres to the mucosa, thus protecting the ulcer from irritation. The therapeutic effects of the drug result from local (i.e., at the ulcer site) rather than systemic activity.

Side effects of sucralfate are rare, with constipation occurring occasionally.

Interactions are possible with sucralfate altering absorption of certain drugs. Avoid giving other drugs within 2h of sucralfate, especially antibiotics and antacids.

Antacids may decrease binding of sucralfate to mucosa, decreasing effectiveness. Separate administration times by 30 min.

## Helicobacter Pylori Treatment

*Helicobacter pylori* bacterial infection plays a major role in the development of gastritis, gastric and duodenal ulceration, and gastric cancer.

*H. pylori* has been treated successfully with multiple-drug regimens (over 14 days). This treatment and possible side effects are discussed in Chapter 17, "Anti-infective Drugs."

# PATIENT EDUCATION

Patients undergoing ulcer therapy should be instructed regarding:

Avoiding cigarette smoking, which seems to decrease the effectiveness of medicines in the healing of duodenal ulcers

Importance of close communication with the physician for possible dosage regulation of other medications taken at the same time

Structuring of environment to reduce stress factors and decrease tension in order to facilitate the healing of ulcers

Not taking antacids within 2h of any other drug

Taking medications on a regular basis and avoiding abrupt withdrawal, which could lead to rebound hypersecretion of gastric acid

Taking sucralfate (Carafate) 1h before meals, on an empty stomach, and not within 2h of any other medicine

Taking misoprostol (Cytotec) with meals and at bedtime with food, and avoiding magnesium products to lessen the incidence of diarrhea

Taking PPIs, esomeprazole (Nexium), lansoprazole (Prevacid), and omeprazole (Prilosec), on an empty stomach; rabeprazole (Aciphex) and pantoprazole (Protonix) can be given without regard to meals.

That self-medication with OTC PPIs is not intended for *immediate relief* of heartburn.

PPIs available as delayed-release dosage forms should *not* be chewed, broken, or crushed.

See Table 16-1 for a listing of the antacids, agents for ulcers and GERD, and protective gastric mucosal medications.

**TABLE 16-1** Antacids, Antiulcer Agents, and Gastric Mucosal Agents

| GENERIC NAME | TRADE NAME | DOSAGE |
|---|---|---|
| **Antacids** (only a sample, many other products are available) | | |
| aluminum hydroxide gel | | Suspension, 600 mg per 5 mL between meals & hs |
| calcium carbonate | Tums | Tabs, 500–2,000 mg orally in two to four divided doses daily |
| aluminum-magnesium combinations with simethicone | Maalox, Gelusil, Mylanta | Suspension, tabs; dose varies with product |
| **Agents for Ulcers and GERD** | | |
| *H₂-Blockers* | | |
| cimetidine | | 300 mg q6h PO |
| | Tagamet HB (OTC) | 200 mg daily BID PO (two weeks max) |
| famotidine | Pepcid | 20 mg BID–40 mg PO tabs at bedtime |
| | | 20 mg IV diluted q12h |
| | Pepcid AC (OTC) | 20 mg daily or 10 mg BID (two weeks max) |
| with calcium carbonate and magnesium hydroxide | Pepcid Complete (OTC) | One to two tabs daily |
| ranitidine | Zantac | 150 mg tabs BID |
| | | 50 mg IV diluted or IM q6–8h |
| | Zantac 75, 150 (OTC) | 150 mg daily or 75 mg BID (two weeks max) |
| *Proton Pump Inhibitors* | | |
| esomeprazole | Nexium | 20–40 mg ac daily SR caps, susp, IV diluted |
| lansoprazole | Prevacid | 15–30 mg ac daily SR caps, |
| | | SoluTab; 30 mg daily IV diluted |
| | Prevacid 24HR (OTC) | 15 mg daily, SR caps (two weeks max) |
| omeprazole | Prilosec | 20–40 mg qAM ac, SR caps, susp |
| | Prilosec OTC | 20 mg daily ac SR tab (two weeks max) |
| with sodium bicarbonate | Zegerid | 20–40 mg ac daily caps, susp |
| | Zegerid OTC | 20 mg ac daily caps (two weeks max) |
| pantoprazole | Protonix | 20–40 mg orally daily SR tabs, susp; 40 mg daily IV diluted |
| rabeprazole | Aciphex | 20 mg daily SR tab |
| *Gastric Mucosal Agents* | | |
| misoprostol | Cytotec | 100–200 mcg four times per day with meals and at bedtime with food |
| sucralfate | Carafate | 1 g four times per day (1h ac and at bedtime), tabs, susp |

# GI ANTISPASMODICS OR ANTICHOLINERGICS

## Dicyclomine

Antispasmodics or anticholinergics help to calm the bowel. Dicyclomine (Bentyl) is an anticholinergic and antimuscarinic agent used for the treatment of irritable bowel syndrome and other functional disturbances of GI motility. GI anticholinergics work by decreasing motility (smooth muscle tone) in the GI tract.

Side effects of dicyclomine, especially in older adults, can include:

- Dry mouth and constipation
- Blurred vision, dizziness, and drowsiness
- Urinary retention (decreases smooth muscle tone in the urinary tract)
- Tachycardia, palpitations
- Confusion (especially in older adults)

Precautions or contraindications of dicyclomine include:

Glaucoma (narrow angle)

Unstable cardiac disease

Obstructive GI disease and ulcerative colitis

Obstructive uropathy (BPH and bladder obstruction)

Myasthenia gravis

Lactation

Interactions of dicyclomine include:

Phenothiazines (decreased antipsychotic effectiveness, increased anticholinergic side effects)

Tricyclic antidepressants (increased anticholinergic side effects)

Opiate agonists (additive depressive effects on GI motility or bladder function)

# AGENTS FOR INFLAMMATORY BOWEL DISEASE

Inflammatory bowel disease (IBD) is a *chronic* condition that causes inflammation in the lining of the GI tract and includes Crohn's disease and ulcerative colitis. One of the main clinical features of this condition is abnormal defecation, which may be predominant constipation or diarrhea. There is no cure for IBD, and treatment strategies focus on symptom control and improvement in the quality of life.

## Salicylates

Mesalamine (Asacol, Rowasa) and the prodrug sulfasalazine (Azulfidine) have chemical structures similar to those of aspirin and exhibit anti-inflammatory activity in the GI tract. They are used in the management of Crohn's disease and ulcerative colitis. These salicylates are all designed to reach the ileum and colon, bypassing the stomach and upper intestines. They are safe for long-term use and are well tolerated in most patients.

Side effects of salicylates (often more frequent and severe with sulfasalazine) can include:

- Anorexia, nausea, vomiting, diarrhea, and dyspepsia
- Abdominal pain, cramps, and bloating (with rectal administration)
- Headache, weakness, dizziness, and rash

Intolerance to sulfasalazine can be minimized by taking the enteric-coated product (Azulfidine EN-tabs).

Precautions and contraindications with sulfasalazine apply to those having:

- Allergy to salicylates
- Allergy to sulfonamides with sulfasalazine (can cause anaphylaxis or asthma attacks)
- Allergy to sulfites (Rowasa enema)

Renal impairment

Hepatic impairment (with sulfasalazine)

Interactions with sulfasalazine include:

Warfarin (increased risk of hemorrhage)

Methotrexate (increased bone marrow suppression)

Cyclosporine (decreased efficacy)

Oral diabetic agents (hypoglycemia)

Folic acid (absorption is inhibited)

## Glucocorticoids

Glucocorticoids (prednisone, prednisolone, hydrocortisone enema) are used to treat moderate to severe *active* forms of IBD in patients who are inadequately controlled with salicylates. The oral steroids do not require direct contact with the inflamed intestinal tissue to be effective. For a detailed discussion on these agents, see Chapter 23, "Endocrine System Drugs."

# ANTIDIARRHEAL DRUGS

Antidiarrheal agents act in various ways to reduce the number of loose stools.

## Bismuth Subsalicylate

Bismuth subsalicylate (e.g., Kaopectate, Pepto-Bismol) has anti-infective and antisecretory properties, a direct mucosal protective effect, and weak antacid and anti-inflammatory effects. Kaopectate brand products have been reformulated several times over the years. Be aware that several formulations of "generic" Kaopectate are still available—check label contents and dosing carefully.

Side effects of bismuth subsalicylate are relatively uncommon at normal doses and include:

- Transient, occasional constipation
- Discoloration of tongue and stool (black color)
- Ringing in ears

Interactions with bismuth subsalicylate are possible, when these agents are administered concurrently with medications such as:

Warfarin (increases bleeding)

Aspirin and methotrexate (increases toxicity)

Quinolones and tetracyclines (decreased bioavailability)

Precautions or contraindications for bismuth subsalicylate include:

Salicylate (including aspirin) hypersensitivity

Children (< 12 years old) or teenagers recovering from chickenpox or influenza (risk of Reye's syndrome)

Coagulation abnormalities and ulcers

Pregnancy and lactation

## PATIENT EDUCATION

Patients treated with bismuth subsalicylate should be instructed regarding:

Avoiding self-medication for longer than 48h or if fever develops

Diet of a bland nature, excluding roughage and including foods containing natural pectin (e.g., apple *without* peelings and without sugar added)

Adequate fluid intake (especially tea *without* sugar for its astringent effect) or intake of oral electrolyte products (i.e., Gatorade, Pedialyte) to prevent dehydration

Contacting the physician immediately if complications develop or condition worsens and if observing blood in stool

Not using bismuth subsalicylate if allergic to salicylates (including aspirin) and in children or teenagers recovering from chickenpox or influenza

Considering all sources of salicylate if taking aspirin or other medications containing salicylate, so that toxic levels are not reached

## Opiate Agonists: Diphenoxylate with Atropine and Loperamide

These products act by slowing *intestinal motility*, thus allowing for more reabsorption of fluid. Lomotil is a product combining diphenoxylate with atropine. It is a Schedule C-V controlled substance. Loperamide (Imodium) is available in various forms; all are OTC products, except for some capsule formulations, which remain prescription-only (see Table 16-2).

Side effects can include:

⚠ Anticholinergic effects with Lomotil (e.g., drying of secretions, blurred vision, urinary retention, lethargy, confusion, or flushing)

⚠ Abdominal distention, nausea, or vomiting with Lomotil or Imodium

Precautions or contraindications include:

Diarrhea caused by infection or poisoning

Fever over 101°F

Young children (under 3 years of age)

Pregnancy

*Clostridium difficile* colitis associated with antibiotics

Obstructive jaundice

Precautions or contraindications apply to older adults.

## PATIENT EDUCATION

Patients taking antidiarrheal drugs should be instructed regarding:

Not exceeding the recommended dosage; short-term (48h) only

Adequate fluid intake and bland diet

Reporting side effects or complications to the physician immediately, or if symptoms persist or worsen

Not taking these medications if diarrhea is caused by infection or food poisoning.

## Probiotics

Probiotics are living microorganisms that can alter a patient's intestinal flora and may provide benefit in numerous GI diseases. The body's naturally occurring gut flora may fall out of balance in a wide range of circumstances, including the use of antibiotics or other drugs, excess alcohol, stress, certain diseases, or exposure to toxic substances.

*Lactobacillus acidophilus* is an acid-producing probiotic bacterium, available in several forms OTC. It is administered orally for the *treatment* of simple uncomplicated diarrhea caused by antibiotics, infection, irritable colon, colostomy, or amebiasis. *Lactobacillus* bacteria help to reestablish normal intestinal flora. The capsules, tablets, powder, or granules may be taken directly or mixed with cereal, food, milk, juice, or water.

Side effects tend to be mild and digestive (gas, bloating) in nature.

Precautions or contraindications for *Lactobacillus* apply to:

Anyone with a high fever; weakened immune system

Those sensitive to milk products or have a lactase deficiency

Long-term use, unless directed by the physician

Patients with prosthetic heart valves or valvular heart disease (risk of bacteremia)

*Saccharomyces boulardii* (Florastor) is a yeast used in dairy fermentation. It is derived from the intestinal microbiota of healthy humans. It is a probiotic often started within three days of antibiotic initiation and continued for three days after discontinuation to *prevent* diarrhea. Probiotic bacteria are also found in yogurt (Activia) and other dairy foods for the replacement of beneficial intestinal tract bacteria.

## Clostridium Difficile Infection

*Clostridium difficile* is one of the most common causes of infectious diarrhea in the United States. Symptoms of *C. difficile* diarrhea (CDD) may include watery diarrhea, nausea, and/or abdominal pain or tenderness. Complications may include sepsis, renal failure, toxic colitis, and death. CDD is caused primarily by the eradication of the native intestinal flora with broad-spectrum antimicrobials and overuse of PPI and $H_2$-blocker therapy.

Oral medications include metronidazole (Flagyl) or vancomycin. See Chapter 17 for more information on these agents. Opiates and antidiarrheal medications may decrease GI motility, thereby increasing toxins in the intestine, so their use *should be avoided.*

## ANTIFLATULENTS

Antiflatulents (e.g., simethicone) are used in the symptomatic treatment of gastric bloating and postoperative gas pains, by helping to break up gas bubbles in the GI tract.

No side effects, precautions and contraindications, or drug interactions have been reported.

## PATIENT EDUCATION

Patients should be instructed to avoid gas-forming foods (e.g., onions, cabbage, and beans).

Precautions or contraindications apply only to infant colic because of limited information on safety in children.

See Table 16-2 for a summary of antispasmodic, inflammatory bowel disease, antidiarrheal, and antiflatulent agents.

**TABLE 16-2** GI Antispasmodic, Inflammatory Bowel Disease, Antidiarrheal, and Antiflatulent Agents

| GENERIC NAME | TRADE NAME | DOSAGE |
|---|---|---|
| **GI Antispasmodics or Anticholinergics** | | |
| dicyclomine | Bentyl | PO 20–40 mg four times per day caps, tabs; IM 20 mg q6h (two days max; switch to PO) |
| **Agents for Inflammatory Bowel Disease** | | |
| *Salicylates* | | |
| mesalamine | Asacol HD | 2 × 800 mg PO TID (up to six weeks), DR tab |
| | Rowasa | 4 g R at bedtime (retain 8 h; use three to six weeks), enema |
| | Canasa | 1,000 mg R at bedtime (retain 1–3 h; use three to six weeks), suppository |
| sulfasalazine | Azulfidine | 500 mg tab or DR tab |
| | Azulrfidine EN-tab | 500 mg–1 g four times per day |
| **Antidiarrheal Agents** | | |
| *Salicylates* | | |
| bismuth subsalicylate | Kaopectate, Pepto-Bismol | Susp, 30 mL or 2 tabs q30–60 min after each BM (max eight doses per day) |
| *Opiate Agonists* | | |
| diphenoxylate with atropine | Lomotil | Sol or tabs, 2.5–5 mg four times per day (max 20 mg per day) |
| loperamide | Imodium caps (Rx) | Sol, tabs, caps; 4 mg initially, 2 mg after each loose BM |
| | Imodium A-D (OTC) | (Rx maximum 16 mg per day; OTC maximum 8 mg per day × 2 days) |
| *Probiotics* | | |
| *Lactobacillus acidophilus* | Lactinex, Bacid | 2 caps, 4 tabs, or 1 pkg granules three or four times per day |
| *Lactobacillus* GG | Culturelle | 1 cap PO BID (continue for one week after discontinuation of antibiotics) |
| *Saccharomyces boulardii* | Florastor | 2 caps PO BID (start within three days of antibiotic; continue for three days after discontinuation) |
| **Antiflatulent** | | |
| simethicone | Mylicon | Liquid, tabs pc, and at bedtime 160–500 mg daily in divided doses |

# LAXATIVES AND CATHARTICS

Laxatives promote evacuation of the intestine and are used to treat constipation. Included in the laxative category are *cathartics,* or *purgatives,* which promote *rapid evacuation* of the intestine and alteration of stool consistency. Laxatives can be subdivided into seven categories according to their action: bulk-forming laxatives, stool softeners, emollients, saline laxatives, stimulant laxatives, osmotic laxatives, and chloride channel activator.

Many OTC laxatives are self-prescribed and overused by a large portion of the population. Prevention and relief of constipation is better achieved through natural methods (e.g., high-fiber diet, adequate fluid intake, good bowel habits, and exercise). Normal frequency of bowel movements varies from daily to several times weekly. When constipation occurs, the cause should be identified before laxatives are used.

## Bulk-Forming Laxatives

Bulk-forming laxatives, also known as fiber supplements (e.g., psyllium, cellulose derivatives, polycarbophil, and bran), soften the stool by absorbing water and increase fecal mass to facilitate defecation. They are the treatment of choice for simple constipation unrelieved by natural methods. These products are available in powders, capsules, tablets, or wafers and *must be dissolved* or *diluted* according to manufacturers' directions (note label). The usual procedure is to take or dissolve the product in one *full glass* of water or juice to be taken orally and followed immediately with another glass of fluid. The proper dosage is administered one to three times per day. Laxative effect is usually apparent within 12–72 h.

Bulk-forming laxatives are the choice for older adults or laxative-dependent patients. They have been useful in maintaining regularity for patients with diverticulosis and in increasing the bulk of stools in patients with chronic watery diarrhea.

Precautions or contraindications for bulk-forming laxatives apply to patients with acute abdominal pain, partial bowel obstruction, dysphagia (difficulty in swallowing), or esophageal obstruction.

## PATIENT EDUCATION

Patients should be instructed regarding:

*Dissolving all bulk-forming products completely* in one full glass of liquid and following that with another glass of fluid to prevent obstruction.

Administering immediately when dissolved, before thickening occurs.

## Stool Softeners

Stool softeners (e.g., docusate) are surface-acting agents that moisten stool through a detergent action and are administered orally. Dosage required to soften stools varies widely depending on the condition and patient response. Stool softeners are the choice for pregnant or nursing women and children with hard, dry stools. The onset of action is usually 12–72 h.

Side effects are rare, with occasional mild, transitory GI cramping or rash.

Precautions or contraindications apply to acute abdominal pain or prolonged use (more than one week) without medical supervision

Caution to avoid stool softeners that also contain stimulant laxatives, for example Peri-Colace, Senokot-S.

## PATIENT EDUCATION

Patients taking stool softeners should be instructed regarding:

Discontinuance with any signs of diarrhea or abdominal pain

Avoiding use for longer than one week without medical supervision

Interaction with mineral oil, which leads to mucosal irritation and systemic absorption of mineral oil

Taking large quantities of fluids to soften stool

Checking package label to be sure no cathartics are included

## Emollients

Emollients promote stool movement through the intestines by softening and coating the stool. Mineral oil may be administered orally and is usually effective in 6–8 h. Mineral oil is sometimes administered rectally as an oil-retention enema (60–120 mL).

Side effects of emollients may include:

- Seepage of oil from rectum, causing anal irritation
- Malabsorption of vitamins A, D, E, and K only with prolonged oral use

Precautions or contraindications for oral mineral oil apply to:

Children under 5 years old

Bedridden, debilitated, or geriatric patients

Patients with dysphagia, gastric retention, or hiatal hernia

Pregnancy

Prolonged use

Concomitant use of stool softeners

## PATIENT EDUCATION

Patients taking mineral oil should be instructed regarding:

Avoiding frequent or prolonged use

Using caution if having trouble swallowing or with aspiration of the oil (potential of lipoid pneumonitis if aspirated); never take mineral oil at bedtime

Interaction with docusate (stool softener), which can facilitate absorption of mineral oil, possibly increasing the risk of toxicity.

## Saline Laxatives

Saline laxatives (e.g., milk of magnesia or citrate of magnesia) promote secretion of water into the intestinal lumen and should be taken only infrequently in single doses. Saline laxatives should not be taken on a regular or repeated basis unless directed by a physician. The onset of action is 0.5–3 h.

Side effects of saline laxatives used for prolonged periods or in overdoses can include:

- Electrolyte imbalance
- CNS symptoms, including weakness, sedation, and confusion
- Edema
- Cardiac, renal, and hepatic complications

Precautions or contraindications apply to:

Long-term use

Heart failure or other cardiac disease

Edema, cirrhosis, or renal disorders

Those taking diuretics

Acute abdominal pain

Colostomy

## PATIENT EDUCATION

Patients taking saline laxatives should be instructed regarding:

Using caution as products of different strengths are available (MOM comes in 400, 800, and 1,200 mg per 5 mL concentrations)

Avoiding saline cathartics with certain medical conditions

Avoiding frequent or regular use of saline cathartics

## Stimulant Laxatives

Stimulant laxatives (e.g., senna, castor oil, and bisacodyl) are cathartic in action, producing strong peristaltic activity, and may also alter intestinal secretions in several ways. Stimulant laxatives are habit forming, and long-term use may result in laxative dependence and the loss of normal bowel function. All stimulant laxatives produce some degree of abdominal discomfort. Their use should be confined to conditions in which rapid, thorough emptying of the bowel is required (e.g., before surgical, proctoscopic, sigmoidoscopic, or radiological examinations, or for emptying the bowel of barium following GI X-rays) or for patients on opioid therapy. Sometimes a combination of oral preparations, suppositories, and/or enemas may be ordered for these purposes. The onset of action is 0.25–8 h, depending on the preparation.

Side effects of stimulant laxatives are common, especially with frequent use, and can include:

- Abdominal cramps or discomfort and nausea (frequent)
  Rectal and/or colonic irritation with suppositories
- Loss of normal bowel function with prolonged use
- Electrolyte disturbances and dehydration with prolonged use
  Discoloration of urine with senna

Precautions or contraindications with stimulant laxatives apply to:

Acute abdominal pain or abdominal cramping—danger of ruptured appendix

Ulcerative colitis

Children and pregnant and lactating women

Long-term use

# PATIENT EDUCATION

Patients taking stimulant laxatives should be given strong warnings against frequent or prolonged use because of the danger of laxative dependence and loss of normal bowel function.
Bisacodyl tablets should not be crushed or chewed or taken within 1h after milk or antacids due to gastric irritation.

## Osmotic Laxatives

Osmotic laxatives such as glycerin, lactulose, polyethylene glycol (PEG), and sorbitol exert an action that draws water from the tissues into the feces and reflexively stimulates evacuation. Response and side effects vary with preparation. Lactulose response may take 24–48 h. Side effects include nausea, vomiting, flatulence, and abdominal cramps. Osmotic laxatives are also used to treat encephalopathy (brain and nervous system damage) in hepatic failure precipitated by GI bleeding and other conditions.

Glycerin rectal suppositories or enemas usually cause evacuation of the colon within 15–60 min. Glycerin may produce rectal irritation or cramping pain. Polyethylene glycol (Miralax) response can be seen in 0.5–3 h; however, two to four days of therapy may be required to produce a bowel movement. Side effects are similar to other drugs in this category; high doses of Miralax can cause electrolyte imbalances (hyponatremia, hypokalemia) with prolonged or excessive use.

## Chloride Channel Activators

Lubiprostone (Amitiza) is a unique oral agent for the treatment of constipation. It increases intestinal fluid secretion by activating specific chloride channels in the intestinal epithelium. Lubiprostone alters stool consistency and promotes regular bowel movements without altering electrolyte balance or producing tolerance. Most patients experience a bowel movement within 24h of the first dose.

Side effects of lubiprostone can include:

- Nausea and diarrhea
- Headache
- Abdominal bloating or pain and flatulence

Precautions or contraindications apply to:

- Severe diarrhea or bowel obstruction
- Renal or hepatic impairment
- Pregnancy and breast-feeding

## PATIENT EDUCATION

Patients with constipation issues should be instructed regarding:

- High-fiber diet to prevent constipation, including roughage (e.g., bran, whole-grain cereals, and fresh fruits and vegetables)
- Adequate fluid intake
- Developing good bowel habits (e.g., regular, at an unrushed time of day)
- Regular exercise to develop muscle tone
- Avoiding any laxative with acute abdominal pain, nausea, vomiting, or fever
- Avoiding laxatives if any medical condition is present, unless prescribed by a physician. Bulk-forming laxatives are safest in the long term.
- Using only the mildest laxatives (e.g., stool softeners) on a short-term, infrequent basis
- Reporting any prolonged constipation, if above measures are ineffective, to a physician for investigation

See Table 16-3 for a summary of laxatives.

**TABLE 16-3** Laxatives

| GENERIC NAME | TRADE NAME | DOSAGE |
|---|---|---|
| **Laxatives** (only a sample, many other products available) | | |
| *Bulk-forming* | | |
| psyllium | Metamucil, Konsyl-D, others | Powder, 1–3 tsp, dissolved in or 2–6 caps taken with full glass of fluid one to three times per day |
| *Stool softener* | | |
| docusate | Colace, others | Oral caps, tabs, liquid 50–300 mg daily |
| *Emollient* | | |
| mineral oil | Fleet Mineral Oil | 15–45 mL PO daily; 60–120 mL R daily |
| *Saline laxative* | | |
| magnesium hydroxide | Milk of Magnesia | Susp, 15–60 mL daily |
| *Stimulant laxatives* | | |
| senna | Senokot | 8.6 mg tab, 1–4 BID or 10–15 mL syrup BID |
| with docusate | Peri-Colace, Senokot-S | 1–2 tabs daily—BID |
| bisacodyl | Dulcolax | 5–15 mg DR tabs, 10 mg Supp |
| | Fleet | 10 mg/30 mL enema |
| *Osmotic laxatives* | | |
| glycerine | Fleet suppository | 1 suppository R PRN |
| lactulose | Enulose | 15–60 mL PO daily (10 g/15 mL) (more frequently for hepatic encephalopathy) |
| polyethylene glycol | Miralax (OTC) GlycoLax (Rx) | 17 g (1 capful) in 4–8 oz liquid daily (OTC—7 days max; Rx—14 days+) |
| sorbitol | | 30–150 mL PO of 70% solution |
| *Chloride channel activator* | | |
| lubiprostone | Amitiza | 8 mcg cap BID with food (IBD with constipation) 24 mcg cap BID with food (constipation) |

*Note:* This is only a representative sample. Others are available. Always read labels carefully, especially with OTC medications.

# ANTIEMETICS

Antiemetics are used in the prevention or treatment of nausea, vomiting, vertigo, or motion sickness. Many different types of products are available, varying in their actions, the condition treated, and route of administration. Prevention is preferred over treatment of established nausea and vomiting.

## Anticholinergics

Motion sickness is mediated by cholinergic and histaminic receptors in the inner ear. For prophylaxis of motion sickness, anticholinergic drugs such as dimenhydrinate (Dramamine) or scopolamine are used. For greatest effectiveness, the Transderm-Scop patch is applied behind the ear 4h before anticipated exposure to motion (do not cut patch) and is effective up to 72h. Dramamine is administered orally 30 min before exposure to motion. Both of these drugs are also available for IM injection in patients who have already developed motion sickness.

Meclizine (Antivert) is an antihistamine used in the prevention and treatment of nausea, vomiting, and/or vertigo associated with motion sickness, and in the symptomatic treatment of vertigo associated with the vestibular system (e.g., Meniere's disease). The onset of action is about 1h, and effects persist 8–24h after a single oral dose. Although meclizine produces fewer adverse anticholinergic effects (dry mouth, confusion, urinary retention) than scopolamine, it can cause drowsiness, but to a lesser degree than dimenhydrinate (Dramamine). It is not recommended for children under age 12.

## Antidopaminergics

Dopamine-receptor antagonists interfere with the stimulation of the chemoreceptor trigger zone (CTZ) in the brain, thereby blocking messages to the GI tract. The most frequently used agents to control nausea and vomiting in this class are prochlorperazine (brand name Compazine, which is no longer marketed) and promethazine (Phenergan), which are related to the phenothiazines, discussed in Chapters 20 and 26, respectively. These drugs are used for symptomatic relief, and their use must be supplemented by restoration of fluid and electrolyte balance, as well as determination of the cause of vomiting.

Antagonism of dopamine receptors in other areas of the brain, including those involved with movement, can lead to extrapyramidal reactions (tremors, difficulty walking, and muscular rigidity), which are common for drugs in this class at high doses. Prochlorperazine shows a high incidence of extrapyramidal reactions, especially in psychiatric patients receiving phenothiazines long term or in children. It is not recommended for children under age 12. *Caution with older adults. Not for long-term use*

For *preoperative* preventive antiemetic effect or *postoperative* treatment for nausea and vomiting, promethazine is usually the drug of choice. Promethazine can be given *deep* IM (50 mg/mL concentration only) or via a central line (25 mg/mL concentration only), but *never* subcutaneously due to the risk of serious tissue injury that may occur. Metoclopramide (Reglan), a dopamine-receptor antagonist unrelated to other agents, is an antiemetic and a stimulant of upper GI motility. It accelerates gastric emptying and intestinal transit. It is used in a variety of GI motility disorders, especially gastric stasis, *short-term* (*up to 12 weeks*) treatment of GERD, and for the prevention (IM/IV only, not oral) of cancer chemotherapy–induced emesis. Extrapyramidal reactions can also occur with metoclopramide.

## Serotonin-Receptor Antagonists

Serotonin is a major neurotransmitter involved in emesis located in the gut. Serotonin-receptor antagonists preferentially block serotonin receptors found centrally in the CTZ and peripherally in the intestines to control emesis. Ondansetron (Zofran) and dolasetron (Anzemet) are used for the prevention and treatment of post-operative nausea and vomiting (PONV) and for the control of chemotherapy-induced nausea and vomiting (CINV).

These agents have fewer side effects (mainly headache, dizziness, drowsiness, and diarrhea) and are usually well tolerated.

Side effects of the antiemetics vary with the drug and dosage, but the most common include:

- Confusion, anxiety, restlessness (especially in older adults)
- Sedation, drowsiness, vertigo, weakness, and headache
- Diarrhea and depression (with Reglan)
- Dry mouth and blurred vision
- Extrapyramidal reactions (involuntary movements), especially in children and older adults with the antidopaminergics

  Cardiac arrhythmias, QT prolongation with high doses or too fast IV administration (see interactions)

Precautions or contraindications with antiemetics apply to:

Children and adolescents (increased risk of movement disorders) with antidopaminergics

Pregnancy and lactation

Debilitated, emaciated, or older adult patients (require reduced dose)

Angle-closure glaucoma

Prostatic hypertrophy

Cardiac arrhythmias or hypertension

Seizure disorders (seizure threshold lowered)

COPD and asthma (Phenergan suppresses cough reflex.)

Interactions of antiemetics resulting in the potentiation of a sedative effect occur with:

CNS depressants, including tranquilizers, hypnotics, analgesics, antipsychotics, alcohol, muscle relaxants (potentiation of sedative effects)

Drugs that prolong QT interval (antiarrhythmics, tricyclic antidepressants, phenothiazines, atypical antipsychotics, "mycin" and quinolone antibiotics, and others)

Metoclopramide (other antiemetics also antagonize the stimulant effects of metoclopramide on the GI tract; promethazine can also increase the risk of extrapyramidal reactions if given with metoclopramide)

SSRI antidepressants (*serotonin syndrome* with promethazine and metoclopramide); serotonin syndrome is caused by excess serotonin release, leading to muscle rigidity, increased temperature, changes in blood pressure, confusion, and eventually death

See Table 16-4 for a summary of antiemetics.

## PATIENT EDUCATION

Patients taking antiemetics should be instructed regarding:

Taking these medications under medical supervision

Determining the cause of nausea and vomiting

Reporting effectiveness or complications

Administering only as directed

Not combining with any other CNS depressants, SSRI antidepressants, alcohol, or muscle relaxants unless prescribed by a physician (e.g., with cancer patients)

## TABLE 16-4 Antiemetics

| GENERIC NAME | TRADE NAME | DOSAGE |
|---|---|---|
| **Antiemetics** | | |
| *Anticholinergics* | | |
| dimenhydrinate | Dramamine (po-OTC; inj-Rx) | 50–100 mg PO or IM, IV q4h PRN for motion sickness (max 400 mg PO, 300 mg IM/IV) |
| meclizine | Dramamine Less Drowsy (OTC) | 25–50 mg daily, 1 h before motion (repeat q24h PRN) |
| | Antivert (Rx) | 25–100 mg in divided doses/Meniere's |
| scopolamine | Transderm-Scop | 72-h patch for motion sickness |
| *Antidopaminergics* | | |
| metoclopramide | Reglan | PO, IM, IV; dose varies with condition |
| prochlorperazine | (Compazine)[a] | 5–10 mg PO, IM, IV, four times per day; 25 mg suppository BID |
| promethazine | Phenergan | Tabs, syrup, deep IM, IV, or suppository |
| | | 12.5–25 mg (never subcu; caution in older adults) |
| *Serotonin-Receptor Antagonists* | | |
| dolasetron | Anzemet | CINV[b]: 100 mg PO; PONV: 12.5 mg IV, 100 mg PO |
| ondansetron | Zofran | CINV: 0.15 mg/kg IV (over 15 min; max 16 mg), 24 mg PO; PONV: 4 mg IM, IV (over 2–5 min), 16 mg PO |

**Note:** This is only a representative sample. Others are available. Always read labels carefully, especially with OTC medications.

[a] This brand name is no longer marketed, but the name is still commonly used.

[b] Dosage with PONV or CINV

# CASE STUDY A

## GASTROINTESTINAL DRUGS

Derek Washington, a 42-year-old male, has called his physician's office to discuss an issue with the advice nurse. He has had diarrhea for the past 24h and would like a recommendation for a medication to relieve this condition.

1. The advice nurse suggests that Derek take some Pepto-Bismol, following the medication's label dosages. Which side effect may occur if he takes an amount over the recommended dosage?
   a. Dehydration
   b. Excessive thirst
   c. Hypoglycemia
   d. Black discoloration of the tongue and stool

2. The advice nurse also checks with Derek to see what other medications he is currently taking. The nurse explains that Derek should be cautious with which of the following when taking Pepto-Bismol?
   a. Iron
   b. Docusate sodium
   c. Warfarin
   d. Ibuprofen

3. Which type of diet will the nurse recommend for Derek while he is taking Pepto-Bismol?
   a. A full liquid diet
   b. A diet high in roughage
   c. A bland diet
   d. A diet that avoids foods with natural pectin

4. The nurse also inquires about Derek's history of allergies to medication. Pepto-Bismol should be avoided in patients who are allergic to which drug?
   a. Penicillin
   b. Salicylates
   c. Naproxen sodium
   d. Glucocorticoids

5. The nurse recommends that Derek take Pepto-Bismol for no longer than:
   a. 48h
   b. 72h
   c. 96h
   d. 1 week

# CASE STUDY B

## GASTROINTESTINAL DRUGS

Helen Hoffmann is taking a bus trip to NYC with a group of friends. She is anxious about the trip because she often experiences motion sickness, so she consults with her physician.

1. Helen's physician suggests a medication to help prevent nausea and vomiting. Which medication will she be most likely to recommend?
   a. Diphenhydramine
   b. Meclizine
   c. Promethazine
   d. Prochlorperazine

2. After further discussion, the physician thinks that Helen would experience less motion sickness with a Transderm-Scop patch. To which area of the body is this patch applied?
   a. On the inner wrist
   b. On the upper arm
   c. Behind the ear
   d. On the anterior abdomen

3. How many hours prior to her bus trip should Helen apply the Transderm-Scop patch to prevent motion sickness?
   a. 1h
   b. 2h
   c. 4h
   d. 8h

4. The physician discusses other options for motion sickness treatment as well. Which medication can be given by IM injection to a patient who already has motion sickness?
   a. Dimenhydrinate
   b. Diphenhydramine
   c. Nexium
   d. Meclizine

5. Which additional instruction regarding the Transderm-Scop patch should the physician give to Helen prior to her bus trip?
   a. The patch will be effective for 24h.
   b. The patch may cause excitability.
   c. Do not cut the patch prior to application.
   d. The patch will work only for motion sickness caused by bus travel.

# CHAPTER REVIEW QUIZ

Match the medication in the first column with the condition in the second column that it is used to treat. Conditions may be used more than once.

| Medication | Condition |
|---|---|
| 1. _____ Nexium | **a.** Diarrhea |
| 2. _____ Antivert | **b.** Flatulence |
| 3. _____ Rowasa | **c.** GERD |
| 4. _____ Lactinex | **d.** Meniere's disease |
| 5. _____ Prevacid | **e.** Nausea and vomiting |
| 6. _____ Transderm-Scop | **f.** Constipation |
| 7. _____ Dulcolax | **g.** Inflammatory bowel disease |
| 8. _____ Simethicone | **h.** Motion sickness |
| 9. _____ Imodium | |
| 10. _____ Phenergan | |

**Choose the correct answer.**

11. With antacids, which of the following applies to administration?

   **a.** Before meals

   **b.** 2h from other medications

   **c.** With Tagamet

   **d.** With milk

12. What is a frequent side effect of calcium carbonate antacids?

   **a.** Diarrhea

   **b.** Fluid retention

   **c.** Constipation

   **d.** Palpitations

13. A patient taking an antispasmodic may experience which side effect?

   **a.** Urinary retention

   **b.** Diarrhea

   **c.** Restlessness

   **d.** Excitability

14. *C. difficile* infection is primarily caused by:

   **a.** Yeast overgrowth in colon

   **b.** Intermittent use of $H_2$ blocker therapy

   **c.** Eradication of native intestinal flora

   **d.** Prolonged use of probiotics

15. When a patient complains of constipation, what is the first action that should be taken?

    **a.** Administer an osmotic laxative.

    **b.** Obtain an abdominal X-ray

    **c.** Administer a bisacodyl tablet with milk.

    **d.** Identify the cause of the constipation.

16. An interaction of an antiemetic drug with another category of drug can result in a potentiation of a sedative effect. What is the second category of drug?

    **a.** Antiarrythmics

    **b.** Antidopaminergics

    **c.** Muscle relaxants

    **d.** Antacids

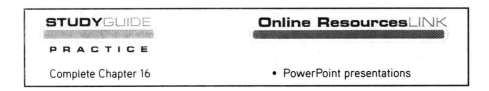

| **STUDY**GUIDE | **Online Resources**LINK |
|---|---|
| **P R A C T I C E** | |
| Complete Chapter 16 | • PowerPoint presentations |

# CHAPTER 19
## ANALGESICS, SEDATIVES, AND HYPNOTICS

## Objectives

*Upon completion of this chapter, the learner should be able to*

1. Compare and contrast the indications and actions of nonopioid, opioid, and adjuvant analgesics, sedatives, and hypnotics

2. List the side effects of the major analgesics, sedatives, and hypnotics

3. Describe the necessary information for patient education regarding interactions and cautions

4. Explain the precautions and contraindications to administration of the CNS depressants mentioned in this chapter

5. Describe actions recently taken by the FDA and manufacturers and the associated impacts on the analgesic drug category

6. Define the Key Terms and Concepts

## Key Terms and Concepts

Adjuvant

Analgesics

Antipyretic

Coanalgesic

Dependence

Endogenous

Endorphins

Hypnotics

Opioid agonists

Opioid antagonists

Paradoxical

Placebo effect

Sedatives

Subjective

Tinnitus

Tolerance

Analgesics, sedatives, and hypnotics depress central nervous system (CNS) action to varying degrees. Some drugs can be classified into more than one category, depending on the dosage. Analgesics are given to relieve pain. Sedatives are given to calm, soothe, or produce sedation. Hypnotics are given to produce sleep.

## ANALGESICS

The most common reason patients seek out medical care is pain. The four most common types of pain reported by the National Center for Health Statistics are lower back, neck, migraine, and facial or jaw pain. Pain is subjective (i.e., it can be experienced or perceived only by the individual person). Health care practitioners can assess a patient's pain by asking the patient to describe the pain and its location, and assess the pain's severity by using validated pain assessment scales.

Pain has both psychological and physiological components. Some persons have a higher pain threshold than others because of conditioning, ethnic background, sensitivity, or physiological factors (e.g., endorphin release). Endorphins are endogenous analgesics produced within the body as a reaction to severe pain or intense exercise (e.g., "runner's high"). Endorphins block the transmission of pain. Endorphin release may be responsible for a placebo effect: relief from pain as the result of suggestion without the administration of an analgesic.

## Opioid Analgesics

Analgesics can be classified as opioid, nonopioid, and adjuvant. Opioids are classified as full or pure agonists, partial agonists, or mixed agonist–antagonists depending on the specific receptors they bind to and their activity at the receptor. Full agonists (e.g., morphine, hydromorphone, oxycodone, and fentanyl) are commonly used because their action is similar to that of opium in altering the perception of pain, and they do not have a ceiling to their analgesic effects, that is, medication level at which there is no enhanced analgesia. The pure agonist opioids will not reverse analgesia like the other classes (e.g., buprenorphine, butorphanol, and nalbuphine).

Due to their potential for abuse and psychological dependence, opioids are classified as controlled substances in the United States and include both the natural opium alkaloids (e.g., morphine and codeine), the semisynthetics (e.g., hydromophone and oxycodone), and the synthetics (e.g., meperidine [Demerol] and fentanyl [Duragesic]). In November 2010, the Food and Drug Administration (FDA) requested a market withdrawal of all products containing propoxyphene (e.g., Darvon and Darvocet), which were linked to cardiac abnormalities and death from overdoses.

Opioids tend to cause tolerance (i.e., a larger dose of opioid is needed to achieve the same level of analgesia) and physiological dependence (i.e., physical adaptation of the body to the opioid and withdrawal symptoms after abrupt drug discontinuation) with chronic use. Addiction or psychological dependence is usually not a problem for patients who require opioids for pain management. The majority of people stop taking opioids when their pain stops. Because of tolerance, the potential for developing dependence, and the potential for developing undesirable side effects, opioids are not used for extended periods except to relieve chronic pain, for example cancer pain, terminal illness, and nonmalignant pain in selected patients who do not benefit from other pain relief methods.

Adequate pain control is important for the terminally ill. Dependence is irrelevant for dying patients and should not be a consideration. More effective pain control can be achieved by combining opioids with nonopioid and adjuvant drugs. Analgesics should be given to terminally ill patients with constant *around-the-clock* pain, with additional "as needed" doses for breakthrough pain, and dosages adjusted to achieve pain relief with an acceptable level of side effects. Around-the-clock dosing prevents pain from developing.

Chronic pain therapy, for example for back pain, sometimes includes the addition of a tricyclic antidepressant or anticonvulsant to the analgesic regimen.

These drugs that enhance analgesic effects are called *adjuvant* analgesics and are explained later in this chapter. This addition can reduce the needed dosage of opioids.

Side effects of opioids can include:

- Sedation
- Confusion, euphoria, restlessness, and agitation
- Headache and dizziness
- Hypotension and bradycardia
- Urinary retention; sexual dysfunction
- Nausea and vomiting (usually resolves within a few days) and constipation (occurs in more than 50% of patients and frequently requires treatment)
- Respiratory depression (appropriate dose titration reduces risk)
- Physical and/or emotional dependence; tolerance
- Blurred vision
- Seizures with large doses
- Flushing, rash, and pruritus (opiate agonists cause histamine release, especially codeine, morphine, and meperidine)

Precautions or contraindications with opioids apply to:

- Head injury (i.e., conditions associated with increased intracranial pressure)
- Cardiac disease (methadone has been associated with QT prolongation, which causes a cardiac arrhythmia that can be fatal in some patients) and hypotension
- CNS depression
- GI, hepatic, renal, and thyroid diseases
- Chronic obstructive pulmonary disease (COPD) and asthma
- Sleep apnea
- Pregnancy and lactation
- Children
- Older adults and debilitated patients
- Driving or operating machinery (may impair mental or physical abilities)
- Addiction prone, suicidal, and alcoholic persons
- Opiate agonist hypersensitivity (can try an opioid from a different chemical class, with close monitoring)
- Abrupt drug discontinuation in patients taking opioids chronically

Interactions include potentiation of the effect of opioids with all CNS depressants, including:

- Psychotropics
- Alcohol

Sedatives and hypnotics

Muscle relaxants

Antihistamines

Antiemetics

Antiarrhythmics or antihypertensives

Preoperatively, an opioid like fentanyl is usually administered parenterally before the start of anesthesia, according to the directions of the anesthesiologist. Meperidine is not recommended for routine use due to a metabolite that may accumulate and cause seizures in patients with kidney disease, although it is useful for the treatment of post-op shivering. Morphine or hydromorphone are commonly used to manage moderate to severe pain due to their longer duration of effect and potency. Hydromorphone is four to eight times more potent than morphine, so caution is necessary to avoid medication errors.

Opioid agonists are available in various strengths, as concentrated oral solutions and in combination products. In January 2011, the FDA announced that drug manufacturers must begin to limit the strength of acetaminophen in *prescription* drug products, which are predominantly combinations of acetaminophen and opioids, to 325 mg per dosage form. This action will help reduce the risk of severe liver injury associated with acetaminophen. Carefully note the product and strength to be administered.

Hydrocodone-containing products, currently a Schedule III controlled substance, were the most commonly prescribed drug in the United States in 2011 (131 million prescriptions for 47 million patients). These products also consistently rank among the most-abused drugs (along with oxycodone) in the United States each year according to the DEA (see Chapter 20). There is a movement by the DEA and the FDA to make hydrocodone-containing products a Schedule II controlled substance, limiting which kind of health care practitioners can write for these products and how many times they can be refilled (see Chapter 1).

## Tramadol

**Tramadol** (Ultram) is a centrally acting synthetic analog of codeine with a dual mechanism of action. It produces analgesia by weak inhibition of norepinephrine and serotonin reuptake and is an opioid receptor agonist. Tramadol has less potential for abuse or respiratory depression (although both may occur) and is currently not classified as a controlled substance on the federal level. However, doses above the normal therapeutic range produce several negative side effects.

Tapentadol (Nucynta) was developed in an attempt to take advantage of the positives associated with tramadol and fewer of its negatives. Tapentadol's mechanism of action does not involve serotonin reuptake, and clinical studies suggest a lower incidence of GI adverse effects. Tapentadol is classified as a Schedule II controlled substance.

**NOTE**

By inhibiting reuptake, the substance (such as serotonin) will be around longer and therefore have a greater effect.

**NOTE**

The opioid antagonist (reversal agent) naloxone (Narcan) is used in the treatment of opioid overdoses and in the operating room, delivery room, and newborn nursery for opiate-induced respiratory depression. Naltrexone (ReVia), a pure opioid antagonist, and sublingual buprenorphine, a partial opioid antagonist, are used separately and together (Suboxone) in the treatment of opioid dependence (see Chapter 20).

Side effects and precautions of tramadol and tapentadol are similar to the opioids listed previously.

Interactions of tramadol and tapentadol occur with:

Monoamine oxidase inhibitors (MAOIs) or neuroleptics (may increase seizure risk)

Carbamazepine (Tegretol) antagonizes tramadol action

Selective serotonin reuptake inhibitors (SSRIs) (especially Paxil, Zoloft), tricyclic antidepressants, and triptans (may cause serotonin syndrome and increase seizure risk)

See Table 19-1 for a summary of the opioid analgesics.

**TABLE 19-1** Opioid Analgesics[a]

| GENERIC NAME | TRADE NAME | DOSAGE | USES/COMMENTS |
|---|---|---|---|
| butorphanol | (Stadol)[b] | 1–4 mg IM, or 0.5–2 mg IV, or 1 mg (one spray) nasal spray q3–4h PRN | Moderate to severe acute pain (e.g., migraine) |
| codeine | | 15–60 mg PO q4h PRN; | Mild to moderate acute, chronic, and cancer pain |
| | | PO 10–20 mg q4–6h PRN (max 120 mg per day) | antitussive dose |
| *with acetaminophen*[c] | Tylenol with Codeine | 15–60 mg codeine PO q4–6h PRN | Max 360 mg codeine and 4 g acetaminophen per day from all sources |
| fentanyl citrate | Actiq (loz.) Fentora (buccal) | PO 200–400 mcg q4–6h PRN; or | Moderate to severe acute, chronic, or cancer pain |
| | (Sublimaze)[b] | 25–100 mcg slow IV/IM | |
| | Duragesic | Transdermal q72h | *Not* for acute pain |
| hydrocodone with acetaminophen[d] *(not available singly)* | Lorcet Lortab Vicodin | PO 2.5–10 mg of hydrocodone (tab or liquid) q4–6h PRN | Moderate acute, chronic, or cancer pain, or antitussive; max 4 g acetaminophen per day |
| hydromorphone | Dilaudid | PO 2–4 mg q4–6h PRN  IM, IV, subcu 0.2–1 mg q2–4h PRN  R 3 mg q6–8h PRN | Moderate to severe acute, chronic, or cancer pain |
| meperidine | Demerol | 50–150 mg PO/IM/IV/subcu, q3–4h PRN | Short-term for moderate to severe *acute* pain |
| methadone | Dolophine Methadose | 2.5–10 mg IM/IV/subcu/PO initially q8–12h PRN; maint. 5–20 mg PO q6–8h PRN | Severe chronic and cancer pain; also for narcotic withdrawal |

(*continued*)

**TABLE 19-1** Opioid Analgesics—*continued*

| GENERIC NAME | TRADE NAME | DOSAGE | USES/COMMENTS |
|---|---|---|---|
| morphine sulfate | | | |
| *immediate release* | morphine | PO 10–30 mg or PR 10–20 mg q3–4h PRN; IV (over 4–5 min); IM/subcu 2.5–15 mg q2–6h PRN | Moderate to severe acute, chronic, or cancer pain |
| *extended release* | MS Contin (tab) | PO, R 15–100 mg q8–12h | Do not crush! OD can be fatal |
| | Avinza (cap) | PO 30 mg q24h (initially, titrate to response) | May open caps and sprinkle contents on applesauce; can give Kadian contents via a gastrostomy tube |
| | Kadian (cap) | PO 10 mg BID or 20 mg QD (initially, titrate to response) | |
| oxycodone | | | |
| *controlled release* | Oxycontin | PO 10–80 mg SR q8–12h | Serious abuse potential, overdose can be fatal; do not crush. |
| *immediate release* | Roxicodone | PO 5–10 mg q6h PRN | Moderate to severe acute, chronic, or cancer pain |
| *with aspirin*[e] | Percodan | PO 1–2 tabs q4–6h PRN | Max 12 tabs per 24h |
| *with acetaminophen*[f] | Percocet | PO 1–2 tabs q4–6h PRN | Max 4 g acetaminophen per day |
| Tramadol | Ultram | PO 50–100 mg q4–6h PRN, max 400 mg daily | Weak opioid analgesic for acute pain, not controlled federally |
| | Ultram ER | PO 100–300 mg daily | Do not crush; for chronic pain |
| *with acetaminophen* | Ultracet | PO 2 tabs q4–6h PRN | Max 8 tabs per day; for acute pain |
| tapentadol | Nucynta | PO 50–100 mg q4–6h PRN | For moderate to severe acute pain |
| | Nucynta ER | PO 50–250 mg SR q12h | For moderate to severe chronic pain; do not crush |

[a]Combination opioid products (check for allergies, especially aspirin combinations).
[b]This brand name is no longer marketed, but the name may still be used.
[c]Tylenol with Codeine tabs contain 300 mg acetaminophen plus codeine:
#2 tab 15 mg codeine, #3 tab 30 mg, #4 tab 60 mg (max acetaminophen dose 4 g per day).
acetaminophen with codeine elixir: 120 mg acetaminophen and 12 mg codeine per 5 mL.
[d]Lortab tabs: 500 mg acetaminophen and 5 mg hydrocodone (subject to reformulation).
Lorcet Plus tabs: 650 mg acetaminophen and 7.5 mg hydrocodone (subject to reformulation).
Lorcet tabs: 650 mg acetaminophen and 10 mg hydrocodone (subject to reformulation).
Vicodan tabs: 300 mg acetaminophen and 5 mg hydrocodone.
Vicodan ES tabs: 300 mg acetaminophen and 7.5 mg hydrocodone.
Vicodin HP tabs: 300 mg acetaminophen and 10 mg hydrocodone.
Lortab elixir: acetaminophen and hydrocodone concentrations vary depending on the manufacturer.
[e]Percodan or Endodan tabs: 325 mg aspirin and 5 mg oxycodone.
[f]Percocet, Roxicet, or Endocet: 325 mg acetaminophen and 5 mg oxycodone. (Other strengths are available.)

# Nonopioid Analgesics

Nonopioid analgesics, many of which are available without prescription as over-the-counter (OTC) medications, are very popular. Therefore, it is extremely important that the health care practitioner be informed and responsible for patient education in this very important area of public health. The lay public needs to become aware of the dangers of self-medication, overdosage, side effects, and interactions, as well as the grave danger of poisoning to children and older adults by inappropriate use of these readily available drugs.

The nonopioids are given for the purposes of relieving mild to moderate pain, fever, and anti-inflammatory conditions, for example arthritis. This group of analgesics is also used as a coanalgesic in severe acute or chronic pain requiring opioids. The salicylates (aspirin) are most commonly used for their *analgesic* and *antipyretic* properties, as well as for their anti-inflammatory action. Other anti-inflammatory drugs, for example ibuprofen, are also used for their analgesic properties. The non-steroidal anti-inflammatory drugs (NSAIDs) are discussed in Chapter 21.

Acetaminophen has analgesic and antipyretic properties but very little effect on inflammation. Aspirin and acetaminophen are frequently combined with opioids (see Table 19-1) or with other drugs for more effective analgesic action. See Table 19-2 for a representative sample of nonopioid analgesics and

**TABLE 19-2** Nonopioid Analgesics and Antipyretics

| GENERIC NAME | TRADE NAME | DOSAGE | COMMENTS |
|---|---|---|---|
| acetylsalicylic acid[a] (ASA, aspirin) | Ecotrin, Ascriptin, Bufferin | 325–650 mg PO or rectal supp q4h PRN; larger doses for arthritis | Administer with milk or food; may cause Reye's syndrome in children and teenagers |
| acetaminophen | Tylenol (OTC) | 325–650 mg PO or rectal supp q4h PRN (max 4 g per day) | No anti-inflammatory action; less effective than ASA for soft tissue pain |
| | Ofirmev (Rx) | 1 g IV q6h PRN or 650 mg q4h PRN (>50 kg) weight-based for less than 50 kg | For mild to moderate pain, fever; for moderate to severe pain with adjunctive opioid analgesics |
| *combinations*[b] ASA and caffeine | Anacin | 2 tabs PO q6h PRN, max 8 per day | |
| ASA, acetaminophen, and caffeine | Excedrin | 2 tabs/caps PO q6h PRN, max 8 per day | Also for the pain of migraine headaches |
| butalbital, caffeine, *with acetaminophen* | Esgic, Fioricet (Rx) | 1–2 tabs/caps PO q4h PRN, max 6 per day | For tension headache or migraine |
| *with aspirin* | Fiorinal (C-III) | | |

[a]Other nonsteroidal anti-inflammatory drugs with analgesic action are listed in Table 21-2.
[b]Representative sample.

antipyretics. There are many other combination analgesic products available OTC. Patients should be instructed to check all ingredients in these combination products because of potentially serious adverse side effects, for example aspirin allergy or acetaminophen contraindications.

## Salicylates and Other NSAIDs

Salicylate analgesic and anti-inflammatory actions are associated primarily with preventing the formation of prostaglandins and the subsequent inflammatory response prostaglandins help to induce. The salicylates, for example aspirin (ASA) and other NSAIDs, are also discussed in Chapter 21.

Side effects of salicylates and other NSAIDs, especially with prolonged use and/ or high dosages, can include:

- Prolonged bleeding time
- Bleeding and frequent bruising
- Gastric distress, ulceration, and bleeding (which may be silent)
- Tinnitus (ringing or roaring in the ears) and hearing loss with overdose
  Hepatic dysfunction
  Renal insufficiency, decreased urine output with sodium and water retention, and renal failure
  Drowsiness, dizziness, headache, sweating, euphoria, and depression
  Rash
- Coma, respiratory failure, or anaphylaxis, which can result from hypersensitivity or overdosage, especially in children (watch for aspirin allergy)
- Gastrointestinal (GI) symptoms, which can be minimized by administration with food or milk or by using an aspirin buffered with antacids or in enteric-coated form
  Poisoning (keep out of reach of children, especially flavored children's aspirin)

Precautions or contraindications for salicylates and other NSAIDs apply to:

GI ulcer and bleeding

Bleeding disorders in patients taking anticoagulants

Asthma

Children younger than 15 with influenza-like illness (because of the danger of Reye's syndrome)

Treatment of pain with NSAIDs after heart surgery

Pregnancy

Lactation

Vitamin K deficiency

Allergy to ASA (occurs in around 2% of the population)

Caution in use of salicylates and other NSAIDs must be taken with:

Anemia

Hepatic disease

Renal disease

Hodgkin's disease

Pre- or postoperative conditions (discontinue five to seven days before elective surgery)

Interactions of salicylates may also occur with NSAIDs and:

Alcohol (may increase potential for ulceration and bleeding)

Anticoagulants (potentiation)

Corticosteroids (gastric ulcer)

Antacids in high doses (decreased effects)

NSAIDs (decreased effects, increased GI side effects)

*Do not give salicylates and NSAIDs together* (unless approved by a physician)

Insulin or oral antidiabetic agents (increased effects; may interfere with certain urinary glucose tests)

Methotrexate (increased effects)

Probenecid (decreased effects)

Antihypertensives: angiotensin-converting enzyme (ACE) inhibitors, beta-blockers and diuretics (decreased effects)

Carbonic anhydrase inhibitors (toxic effects, e.g., Diamox)

## Acetaminophen

Acetaminophen (Tylenol) is used extensively in the treatment of mild to moderate pain and fever. It has very little effect on inflammation. However, acetaminophen has fewer adverse side effects than the salicylates (e.g., does not cause gastric irritation or precipitate bleeding). Therefore, it is sometimes used only for its analgesic properties in treating the chronic pain of arthritis so that the salicylate dosage may be reduced to safer levels with fewer side effects in these patients.

Side effects of acetaminophen are rare, but large doses can cause:

Severe liver toxicity

Renal insufficiency (decreased urine output)

Rash or urticaria

Blood dyscrasia

Caution must be used with frequent acetaminophen use and alcohol ingestion because of potential liver damage. Caution must also be used with pregnancy and breast-feeding.

Contraindicated with hypersensitivity to acetaminophen or any component of the combination product.

Recently there have been major changes in acetaminophen liquid concentrations for pediatrics and lower dosing limits for adults. These *voluntary* changes are being implemented by manufacturers of acetaminophen and are designed to lower the risk of accidental overdoses when too much acetaminophen is ingested, resulting in liver toxicity. The traditional 80 mg/0.8 mL and 80 mg/1 mL concentrated infant drops are to be phased out, and all single-ingredient acetaminophen liquid products for pediatric patients are to be transitioned to a less concentrated children's formulation of 160 mg/5 mL and to include standardized dosing devices, such as oral syringes.

For adults, some manufacturers are lowering the maximum daily dose on single-ingredient acetaminophen products from 4,000 mg per day to 3,000 mg per day. Since these changes are voluntary, there is actually a greater potential for dosing confusion and errors during this transition period. It is imperative that parents, patients, and caregivers read the drug facts label for each specific product carefully to identify the concentration, recommended dosing, and directions for use of that particular product.

# Adjuvant Analgesics

These drugs were originally intended for the treatment of conditions other than pain. Adjuvant analgesics may enhance the analgesic effect with opioids and nonopioids, produce analgesia alone, or reduce the side effects of analgesics. Nerve pain (neuropathic pain) can be caused by certain disease states (diabetic neuropathy), infections (postherpetic neuralgia), and medications (certain chemotherapeutic agents and antiretrovirals). Fibromyalgia is a condition characterized by chronic, widespread musculoskeletal pain; muscle tenderness; sleep disturbances; and profound fatigue.

Both neuropathic pain and fibromyalgia may not be relieved by the pain medications discussed earlier. Two classes commonly used for analgesia in these conditions include anticonvulsants and specific classes of antidepressants. Another agent, lidocaine, is available topically in a patch (Lidoderm) and may be especially effective to treat nerve pain and other types of localized pain while avoiding the adverse effects of oral or parenterally administered medications.

# Tricyclic Antidepressants

Tricyclic antidepressants are used in the treatment of fibromyalgia and nerve pain associated with herpes, arthritis, diabetes, and cancer; migraine or tension headaches; insomnia; and depression. Often, the patient will describe the pain as "burning." Tricyclic antidepressant actions are associated with increasing available norepinephrine and serotonin, which blocks pain transmission. Drugs in this class used commonly for pain include amitriptyline, desipramine, and nortriptyline. Allow two to three weeks to see therapeutic effects.

Side effects of tricyclic antidepressants (more so with amitriptyline) can include:

- Dry mouth, urinary retention, delirium, and constipation
- Sedation (take at bedtime)

⬇ Orthostatic hypotension

⬇ Tachyarrhythmias

Heart block in cardiac patients

The degree of side effects varies with each antidepressant. Side effects may be additive with opioids (e.g., increased constipation, hypotension, and sedation).

Caution must be used with tricyclics if used with prostatic hypertrophy, urinary retention, increased intraocular pressure, and glaucoma.

Precautions or contraindications for tricyclics apply to hypersensitivity and recovery phase of myocardial infarction.

See Chapter 20 for more information on the tricyclic antidepressants.

## Serotonin Norepinephrine Reuptake Inhibitors

Duloxetine (Cymbalta) and venlafaxine (Effexor XR) are antidepressants that inhibit the reuptake of both serotonin and norepinephrine. They do not affect histamine or muscarinic receptors like the tricyclics; therefore, anticholinergic side effects are not present. The SNRI antidepressants are used to treat diabetic neuropathy and fibromyalgia. Milnacipran (Savella), an SNRI with antidepressant activity, is indicated only for fibromyalgia.

Side effects of SNRIs include sleep disturbance, headache, nausea, stomach pain, diarrhea, constipation, dizziness, and sweating. Venlafaxine has the potential to increase blood pressure and heart rate.

Precautions or contraindications apply to narrow-angle glaucoma, hepatic (duloxetine, venlafaxine) or renal (milnacipran) impairment, abrupt discontinuation, patients with a history of suicidal ideation or behaviors, and substantial alcohol use.

Interactions with all SNRIs and serotonergics (such as MAOIs or SSRIs) may result in a serotonin syndrome that is characterized by a rapid development of hyperthermia, hypertension, rigidity, autonomic instability, and mental status changes that can include coma and delirium. Milnacipran has fewer interactions than the other SNRIs.

## Anticonvulsants

Anticonvulsants (i.e., Neurontin and Tegretol), like tricyclic antidepressants, are commonly used for the management of nerve pain associated with neuralgia, herpes zoster (shingles), and cancer. Anticonvulsant therapy is implemented when the patient describes the pain as "sharp," "shooting," "shock-like pain," or "lightning-like."

Gabapentin (Neurontin) is generally considered a first-line *anticonvulsant* for neuropathic pain therapy, followed by carbamazepine (Tegretol) and lamotrigine (Lamictal). Carbamazepine is also indicated for trigeminal neuralgia (also known as tic douloureux), symptoms that include episodes of facial pain, often accompanied by painful spasms of facial muscles.

Pregabalin (Lyrica), a compound that is chemically and structurally similar to gabapentin, is a second-generation anticonvulsant approved by the FDA for use in fibromyalgia, diabetic neuropathy, and postherpetic neuralgia. Pregabalin has been designated as a Schedule V controlled substance because of its potential for abuse and dependence.

Side effects of anticonvulsants can include:

- Sedation, dizziness, and confusion
- Nausea, vomiting, constipation, and anorexia
- Ataxia and unsteadiness
- Hepatitis (not Lyrica)
- Rash, Stevens–Johnson syndrome (Lamictal—start low, slow titration upward)
- Bone marrow suppression
- Nystagmus, diplopia (double vision), and blurred vision
- Gingivitis (gabapentin)
- Weight gain and peripheral edema (pregabalin)

Caution must be used with anticonvulsants if used with allergies, hepatitis, cardiac disease, and renal disease.

CAUTION    Do not confuse *Lamictal* (anticonvulsant) with Lamisil (antifungal).

Precautions or contraindications with anticonvulsants include:

- Hypersensitivity
- Psychiatric conditions (increased risk of suicidal ideation and behavior)
- Pregnancy
- SA (sinoatrial) and AV (atrioventricular) block (Tegretol)
- Hemolytic disorders (Tegretol)
- Abrupt discontinuation

Interactions of anticonvulsants occur with:

- Alcohol (decreased effects)
- Antacids (decreased effects) (Neurontin)
- Antineoplastics (decreased effects) (Tegretol)
- CNS depressants (decreased effects) (Tegretol)
- Folic acid (decreased effects) (Lamictal)
- ACE inhibitors and the antidiabetic agents Actos and Avandia with Lyrica (increased risk of angioedema)
- Antiretrovirals (increased or decreased effects) with Lamictal and Tegretol

# LOCAL ANESTHETICS

The lidocaine patch (Lidoderm) is approved for the management of postherpetic neuralgia, although it can provide significant analgesia in other forms of neuropathic pain, including diabetic neuropathy and musculoskeletal pain such as osteoarthritis and lower back pain. Topical lidocaine provides pain relief through a peripheral effect and generally has little if any central action. The penetration of topical lidocaine into the intact skin is sufficient to produce an analgesic effect, but less than the amount necessary to produce anesthesia.

*The lidocaine patch must be applied to the intact skin.* Patches may be cut into smaller sizes with scissors before the removal of the release liner. To reduce the potential for serious adverse effects, patches are worn only once for up to 12h within a 24h period and then removed. It may take up to two weeks to achieve the desired outcomes.

Side effects of the lidocaine patch, local in nature, are generally mild and transient and include:

- Erythema, edema, and hives
- Allergic reactions

Precautions or contraindications for the lidocaine patch apply to:

Sensitivity to local anesthetics

Hepatic disease

Nonintact skin

Pregnancy, breast-feeding, and pediatric use

Handling and disposal to prevent access by children or pets

Drug interactions of the lidocaine patch occur with:

Antiarrhythmic drugs such as mexiletene

Local anesthetics

See Table 19-3 for a summary of adjuvant analgesics.

**NOTE**

Sometimes a local vasoconstricting agent such as epinephrine is given in conjunction with a local anesthetic injection such as lidocaine to further help localize the effect and thereby prolong the duration of the effect.

# ANTIMIGRAINE AGENTS

Migraine is the most common neurovascular headache and may include nausea, vomiting, and sensitivity to light or noise. Migraines (and most other forms of headache) respond best when treated early. Simple analgesics (see Table 19-2), NSAIDs (see Chapter 21), and opioid analgesics can be effective, especially if they are taken at the initial sign of migraine.

## Serotonin Receptor Agonists (SRAs)

For those patients unresponsive to the aforementioned treatments, serotonin agonists were developed based on the observation that serotonin levels decrease, while vasodilation and inflammation of blood vessels in the brain increase, as the migraine symptoms worsen during an attack. SRAs are also effective in treating the nausea and vomiting associated with migraines because serotonin receptors are also found in the GI tract.

**TABLE 19-3** Adjuvant Analgesics and Local Anesthetic

| GENERIC NAME | TRADE NAME | DOSAGE[a] | COMMENTS |
|---|---|---|---|
| **Antidepressants** | | | |
| *Tricyclics* | | | |
| amitriptyline | (Elavil)[b] | PO 10–150 mg at bedtime | Use with caution in the older adults |
| nortriptyline | Pamelor | PO 10–150 mg at bedtime | Both of these are less likely to cause |
| desipramine | Norpramin | PO 10–150 mg at bedtime | certain side effects vs. amitriptyline |
| *SNRIs[c]* | | | |
| duloxetine | Cymbalta | PO 60–120 mg daily | |
| milnacipran | Savella | Titrate PO to 50–100 mg BID | For fibromyalgia only |
| venlafaxine | Effexor XR | PO 75–225 mg daily | |
| **Anticonvulsants** | | | |
| carbamazepine | Tegretol | PO 200–600 mg BID | Especially for trigeminal neuralgia; monitor serum levels periodically |
| gabapentin | Neurontin | PO 600–3,600 mg per day divided doses three to four times per day | For nerve pain, especially postherpetic neuralgia |
| lamotrigine | Lamictal | PO 25–200 mg BID | Slow titration to avoid rash |
| pregabalin | Lyrica | PO 150–600 mg per day in two to three divided doses | Slow titration to avoid rash; for fibromyalgia, diabetic neuropathy, and postherpetic neuralgia |
| **Local Anesthetic** | | | |
| lidocaine | Lidoderm | 1–3 patches 5% daily (may be cut into smaller sizes) | For postherpetic neuralgia (on 12h/off 12h) |

[a]All adjuvants should be started at the lower end of the dosage range and titrated upward in small increments weekly according to the clinical response.
[b]This brand name is no longer marketed, but the name is still commonly used.
[c]Serotonin norepinephrine reuptake inhibitors.

The first "triptan" approved was sumatriptan (Imitrex), followed by six others. SRAs are indicated for the acute treatment of migraines in adults and are not FDA approved for the prophylactic management of migraine headaches. Nasal spray formulations may be useful if the patient has nausea and vomiting or cannot swallow tablets. Individual responses to triptans vary; patients who do not respond to one triptan may respond to another.

Side effects of SRAs include:

- Malaise, fatigue, dizziness, and drowsiness
- Nausea, vomiting, and diarrhea
  Asthenia, tingling, paresthesias, and flushing
  Pain or pressure in the chest, neck, or jaw
- Arrhythmias, angina, palpitations, myocardial infarction, and cardiac arrest

Precautions or contraindications with SRAs apply to:

Patients with cerebrovascular or cardiovascular disease

Uncontrolled hypertension

Peripheral vascular disease

Hepatic or renal disease (dose adjustments may be needed)

Older adults (who are more likely to have decreased hepatic function and more pronounced blood pressure increases and are at risk for coronary artery disease)

Pregnancy and lactation

Children

Drug interactions of SRAs occur with:

Ergot alkaloids (i.e., methylergonovine; additive vasospastic effects)

MAOIs elevate the plasma levels of *most* triptans (do not use within two weeks of discontinuing the use of the MAOI)

Most antidepressants potentiate the effects of serotonin (including SSRIs and tricyclics) and may result in serotonin syndrome (mental status changes, diaphoresis, tremor, hyperreflexia, and fever) when used in combination

Macrolide antibiotics, antiretroviral protease inhibitors, and "azole" antifungals with eletriptan (increased plasma levels) (do not use within at least 72h of each other).

See Table 19-4 for information on antimigraine agents.

## TABLE 19-4 Antimigraine Agents

| GENERIC NAME | TRADE NAME | DOSAGE FORMS | INITIAL DOSE ADULT | REPEAT TIME (HOURS) | DAILY MAXIMUM DOSE (MG) |
|---|---|---|---|---|---|
| eletriptan | Relpax | Tablet | 20–40 mg | 2 | 40 |
| frovatriptan | Frova | Tablet | 2.5 mg | 2 | 7.5 |
| rizatriptan | Maxalt | Tablet | 5–10 mg | 2 | 30 |
| | Maxalt-MLT | OD tablet | 5–10 mg | 2 | 30 |
| sumatriptan | Imitrex | subcu | 4 mg, 6 mg | 1 | 12 |
| | | Nasal | 5–20 mg | 2 | 40 |
| | | Tablet | 25–100 mg | 2 | 200 |
| zolmitriptan | Zomig | Tablet | 2.5–5 mg | 2 | 10 |
| | Zomig-ZMT | OD tablet | 2.5–5 mg | 2 | 10 |
| | Zomig | Nasal | 5 mg | 2 | 10 |

**OD,** orally disintegrating tablet.
**Note:** Representative sample; other products are available.

# SEDATIVES AND HYPNOTICS

Sedatives and hypnotics are medications used to promote sedation in smaller doses and promote sleep in larger doses. Insomnia is one of the most prevalent sleep disorders, with symptoms occurring in approximately 33% to 50% of the U.S. adult population. The prevalence of chronic insomnia is higher in women and older people. The sedative-hypnotics discussed in this section are classified as benzodiazepines (BZDs) and nonbenzodiazepines (non-BZDs). Some psychotropic drugs like trazodone and mirtazapine (see Chapter 22) and some antihistamines (see Chapter 26 and discussed next) are also used as sedative-hypnotics.

*Antihistamines*, for example diphenhydramine (Benadryl, Nytol, Sominex) and doxylamine (Unisom), have an extended half-life, remaining in the system longer. Because of slower metabolism and impaired circulation, the older or debilitated patient is particularly susceptible to *side effects*, such as blurred vision, dizziness, hypotension, confusion, and decreased coordination. These effects can continue for a longer time, resulting in "morning-after" problems. Tolerance can develop to sleep-inducing effect but not side effects. Therefore, antihistamines are not as effective as other available sedative-hypnotics.

None of these medications should be used for extended periods of time (> 10 days) except under close medical supervision because of the potential for psychological and physical dependence. In addition, these medications depress the REM (rapid eye movement, or dream) phase of sleep, and withdrawal after prolonged use can result in a severe rebound effect with nightmares and hallucinations. Abrupt withdrawal of hypnotics, even after short-term therapy, for example one week, may result in rebound insomnia. Therefore, gradual reduction of dosage is indicated.

Before starting pharmacological treatment, patients should be encouraged to use nondrug interventions to combat insomnia. These include exercise during the day; avoiding daytime naps; avoiding heavy meals and activating medications near bedtime; and warm milk, back rubs, soft music, relaxation techniques, and other calming influences. In addition, avoidance of caffeine and alcohol should be stressed. Alcohol may help to initiate sleep but results in early awakening.

*Barbiturates* are rarely used now as sedative-hypnotics because of the many serious, potentially dangerous *side effects,* especially *CNS depression.* Phenobarbital is still used in the treatment of seizure disorders (see Chapter 22). However, there are many other safer and more effective hypnotics available. Therefore, the use of barbiturates for sedation is restricted to specific, limited circumstances in which the patient can be closely monitored (i.e., Brevital for general anesthesia induction and maintenance).

## Benzodiazepines and Nonbenzodiazepines

Benzodiazepines (BZDs) like temazepam (Restoril) and nonbenzodiazepines (non-BZDs) like zolpidem (Ambien) have supplanted barbiturates as sedative-hypnotics and have less potential for abuse. However, withdrawal effects are observed after long-term use, and *respiratory depression* (when taken with alcohol) can be potentially fatal. As mentioned earlier, the cause of insomnia should be established and underlying factors should be treated before a hypnotic is prescribed. Only short-term use (7–10 days) is recommended for most agents. Like BZDs, non-BZDs are classified as controlled substances due to the possibility of physical and psychological dependence.

Side effects of all the sedative-hypnotics can include:

- Daytime sedation, confusion, and headache—hangover
- Increased risk of falls (especially in older adults or with long-acting hypnotics)
- Dependence or withdrawal symptoms
- Amnesia, hallucinations, and bizarre behavior (may occur more often with triazolam [Halcion] than with other benzodiazepines)

  Metallic aftertaste with Lunesta
- Sleepwalking and engaging in complex tasks (i.e., "sleep eating," "sleep driving," and "sleep-sex")

Precautions or contraindications for all the sedative-hypnotics apply to:

Hypersensitivity

Severe liver impairment

Coadministration of azole antifungals or protease inhibitors with triazolam

Severe renal impairment

Porphyria (with BZDs)

Abrupt discontinuation

Older adults

Debilitated patients

Addiction-prone patients

Renal impairment

Liver impairment

Depressed and mentally unstable people

Individuals who have suicidal ideation or behavior

Pregnancy and lactation

Children

COPD and sleep apnea

Interactions of all the sedative-hypnotics with the following drugs can be dangerous and potentially fatal:

Psychotropic drugs

Alcohol

Muscle relaxants

Antiemetics

Antihistamines

Analgesics

# Melatonin Receptor Agonist

Ramelteon (Rozerem) is the first FDA-approved prescription medication that acts on melatonin receptors, mimicking the actions of melatonin to trigger sleep onset. As a result of this mechanism of action, dependence and abuse potential are eliminated, and ramelteon is not classified as a controlled substance.

Ramelteon works quickly, generally inducing sleep in less than 1h (give within 30 min of going to bed with a high-fat meal or snack). There have been no studies comparing the effectiveness of ramelteon against other hypnotics or even against melatonin supplements (see Table 11-3 for information regarding melatonin). Dose reductions are not required in older adults; however, ramelteon should be used with caution in patients with hepatic impairment.

The use of ramelteon is contraindicated with fluvoxamine (Luvox), which inhibits the metabolism of ramelteon. Do not use ramelteon with melatonin due to the potential for additive sedative effects.

See Table 19-5 for a summary of the sedatives and hypnotics.

**TABLE 19-5** Sedatives and Hypnotics (Use Hypnotics Short Term Only)

| GENERIC NAME | TRADE NAME | DOSAGE | COMMENTS |
|---|---|---|---|
| **Benzodiazepines** | | | |
| temazepam | Restoril | 7.5–30 mg PO at bedtime | Intermediate onset, duration |
| triazolam | Halcion | 0.125–0.25 mg PO at bedtime | Can cause amnesia, hallucinations, bizarre behavior, rapid onset, and short duration |
| **Nonbenzodiazepines** | | | |
| eszopiclone | Lunesta | PO 1–3 mg at bedtime | Rapid onset; not limited to short-term use |
| zolpidem | Ambien[a] | 5–10 mg PO at bedtime | Rapid induction 30 min; short half-life (less than 3h); CR not limited to short-term use |
| | Ambien CR[a] | PO 6.25–12.5 mg at bedtime | |
| | Intermezzo | SL 1.75 or 3.5 mg one per night | For middle-of-the-night awakening with 4h left before planned wake time |
| zaleplon | Sonata | PO 5–10 mg at bedtime | Rapid onset, very short half-life |
| **Melatonin Receptor Agonist** | | | |
| ramelteon | Rozerem | PO 5–10 mg within 30 min of bedtime | Not limited to short-term use; not a controlled substance |

**Note:** [a]Recent FDA warning suggests limiting dose in females to 5 mg regular release and 6.25 mg controlled release due to prolonged levels in blood and slower elimination than males.

# PATIENT EDUCATION

Patients taking analgesics, sedatives, or hypnotics should be instructed regarding:

Potential for physical and psychological dependence and tolerance with opioids, sedatives, and hypnotics

Taking only limited doses for short periods of time, *except* to relieve pain in terminal illness (in terminal cases, analgesics should be given on a regular basis around the clock to prevent or control pain)

Caution with interactions; *not* taking any medications (except under close medical supervision) that potentiate CNS depression (e.g., psychotropics, *alcohol*, muscle relaxants, antihistamines, antiemetics, cardiac medications, and antihypertensives)

Serious potential side effects with prolonged use or overdose of opioids, sedatives, and hypnotics (e.g., oversedation, dizziness, headache, confusion, agitation, nausea, constipation, urinary retention, and *potentially fatal* respiratory depression, bradycardia, or hypotension)

*Tolerance* with prolonged use, with increasingly larger doses required to achieve the same effect

Potential for overdose of sedatives or hypnotics and paradoxical reactions with older adults (e.g., confusion, agitation, hallucinations, and hyperexcitability)

Withdrawal after prolonged use of sedatives and hypnotics, possibly leading to rebound effects with nightmares, hallucinations, or insomnia

Mental alertness and physical coordination impairment, causing accidents or falls

Caution regarding OTC analgesic and sleep aid combinations and checking ingredients on the label; being aware of possible side effects with those containing aspirin (e.g., gastric distress or bleeding)

Not discontinuing abruptly

Proper storage and disposal of these medications

The website www.pain-topics.org is a very good noncommercial resource for health care professionals and their patients, providing open access to clinical news, information, research, and education for evidence-based pain-management practices.

# CASE STUDY A

## ANALGESICS

Seventy-two-year-old Maureen O'Malley is in the recovery room after just having undergone a right total hip replacement for severe arthritis.

1. The recovery room nurse will administer which category of medication *first* to relieve Maureen's pain?
   a. Hypnotic
   b. Sedative
   c. Analgesic
   d. Anti-inflammatory

2. After administering an opioid analgesic, the nurse should observe Maureen for which side effect?
   a. Constipation
   b. Respiratory depression
   c. Abdominal pain
   d. Hypoglycemia

3. The best method to assess Maureen's response to the analgesic is to observe:
   a. Her facial expression
   b. Her respiratory rate
   c. The rating of her pain on a pain scale
   d. The ability to open her eyes

4. While reviewing Maureen's medication orders, the nurse keeps in mind that which additional drug can cause potentiation of the opioid?
   a. Anti-inflammatory
   b. Stool softener
   c. Gastric ulcer medication
   d. Muscle relaxant

5. The nurse administering an opioid to Maureen will use extreme caution if she has a history of:
   a. Arthritis
   b. Allergy to penicillin
   c. COPD
   d. Cataracts

# CASE STUDY B

## HYPNOTICS

Sanjay Rudip has been experiencing insomnia for the past six weeks. At his annual physical, Sanjay reports to his physician that he saw a commercial for Lunesta (eszopiclone) and wants to know if this medication is right for him.

1. The physician explains to Sanjay that hypnotic medications should not be used for extended amounts of time except under close medical supervision. What is the primary reason for this?
   a. Loss of functioning due to an inability to stay awake during the day
   b. An increase in REM sleep as a withdrawal symptom
   c. Risk of cardiac arrest
   d. Physical and psychological dependence

2. Eszopiclone falls into which category of sedatives or hypnotics?
   a. Nonbenzodiazepine
   b. Benzodiazepine
   c. Melatonic receptor agonist
   d. Antihistamine

3. The physician discusses possible interactions of other drugs and hypnotic medications with Sanjay. Which category of drug may potentiate CNS depression when taken in conjunction with a hypnotic and should therefore be avoided?
   a. Anti-infective
   b. Antihistamine
   c. Anticoagulant
   d. Glaucoma

4. The physician warns Sanjay that when taking a hypnotic, he may develop tolerance. What does this mean?
   a. The body will release its own analgesia.
   b. A larger dose will be required over time to achieve the same effect.
   c. Sanjay will experience a lower pain threshold in the future.
   d. Relief from pain will be as a result of a suggestion without the actual administration of a medication.

5. A side effect of prolonged use of a hypnotic is
   a. Dizziness
   b. Tachycardia
   c. Urinary incontinence
   d. Asthma

# CHAPTER REVIEW QUIZ

Match the medication in the first column with the classification in the second column. Classifications may be used more than once.

| Medication | Condition |
|---|---|
| 1. amitripytline | **a.** Antitussive |
| 2. Vicodin | **b.** Opioid antagonist |
| 3. Imitrex | **c.** Opioid analgesic with aspirin |
| 4. methadone | **d.** Tricyclic antidepressant (adjuvant) |
| 5. Percodan | **e.** Opioid analgesic with acetaminophen |
| 6. Duragesic | **f.** Nonopioid analgesic (not controlled) |
| 7. fentanyl | **g.** Anticonvulsant (adjuvant analgesic) |
| 8. codeine | **h.** Synthetic analgesic for acute pain |
| 9. Narcan | **i.** Opioid analgesic and narcotic withdrawal |
| 10. Tegretol | **j.** Transdermal analgesic for chronic pain |
| | **k.** Antimigraine |

**Choose the correct answer.**

11. Which medication is used to treat opiate-induced respiratory depression?

    **a.** Butorphanol

    **b.** Naloxone

    **c.** Methadone

    **d.** Oxycodone

12. Nonopioid analgesics are commonly obtained by which method?

    **a.** From a pharmacist

    **b.** Over the counter

    **c.** With a prescription

    **d.** From a mail-order company

13. Salicylates are most commonly used for which properties?

    **a.** Analgesic or antipyretic

    **b.** Analgesic only

    **c.** Anti-inflammatory

    **d.** Antitussive

14. Which group of medications is used as a coanalgesic in severe or chronic pain?

    **a.** Opioids

    **b.** Nonopioids

    **c.** Hypnotics

    **d.** Sedatives

15. GI symptoms experienced from taking salicylates can be minimized by taking the medication by which of the following methods?

    **a.** With a small glass of water

    **b.** Divided doses

    **c.** Once-a-day dosing

    **d.** Enteric-coated pills

---

**STUDY**GUIDE

**P R A C T I C E**

Complete Chapter 19

**Online Resources**LINK

• PowerPoint presentations

# CHAPTER 20

## PSYCHOTROPIC MEDICATIONS, ALCOHOL, AND DRUG ABUSE

## Objectives

*Upon completion of this chapter, the learner should be able to*

1. Categorize the most commonly used psychotropic medications according to the following classifications: CNS stimulants for promoting wakefulness and treating attention-deficit hyperactivity disorder (ADHD), antidepressants, antimanic agents for bipolar disorders, anxiolytics, antipsychotic medications, and tranquilizers

2. List the purposes, actions, side effects, interactions, and precautions and contraindications for psychotropic medications in common use

3. Describe the physiological effects of prolonged alcohol use

4. Explain the treatment of acute and chronic alcoholism

5. Compare and contrast drug addiction and habituation

6. Describe the effects of commonly used illegal drugs

7. List the responsibilities of a health care practitioner in combating drug abuse

8. Define the Key Terms and Concepts

## Key Terms and Concepts

Addiction

Antidepressant

Antipsychotic

Anxiolytics

Ataxia

Atypical antipsychotics

Bipolar disorders

Chemical dependency

Extrapyramidal

Heterocyclic

Monamine oxidase inhibitors (MAOIs)

Neurotransmitters

Psychotropic

Selective norepinephrine reuptake inhibitors (SNRIs)

Selective serotonin reuptake inhibitors (SSRIs)

Tardive dyskinesia

Tricyclics

Psychotropic refers to any substance that acts on the mind. Psychotropic medications are drugs that can exert a therapeutic effect on a person's mental processes, emotions, or behavior. Drugs used for other purposes can also have psychotropic effects. Examples of other medications that affect mental functioning are anesthetics, analgesics, sedatives, hypnotics, and antiemetics, which are discussed in other chapters.

Psychotropic medications can be classified according to the purpose of administration. The five classes are central nervous system (CNS) stimulant, antidepressant, anxiolytic, antimanic, and antipsychotic medications. Psychotropic medications are frequently prescribed concurrently with psychotherapy or professional counseling.

# CNS STIMULANTS

CNS stimulant medications are given for the purpose of promoting CNS functioning. Drugs in this category include caffeine, amphetamine/methylphenidate preparations, and the wakefulness-promoting agents.

## Caffeine

Fatigue and drowsiness are part of everyday life for millions of people. The only over-the-counter (OTC) drug proven safe and effective in helping fight fatigue and drowsiness is caffeine (at doses of 100–200 mg not more often than every 3–4h), found in products like NoDoz and Vivarin. One prescription-only drug in this category, caffeine citrate (Cafcit), has been used in the treatment of neonatal apnea to stimulate the CNS's respiratory drive.

Prolonged, high intake of caffeine in any form may produce tolerance, habituation, and psychological dependence. Physical signs of withdrawal such as headaches, irritation, nervousness, anxiety, and dizziness may occur upon abrupt discontinuation of the stimulant. Excessive consumption of caffeine (especially when taken with alcohol or other drugs) can lead to life-threatening irregular heartbeats, heart attacks, and seizures. A rising number of patients, many of them young students, are being treated in emergency rooms for complications related to the consumption of highly caffeinated energy drinks.

Since caffeine crosses the placenta and is also distributed into the milk of nursing women, most clinicians recommend that those who are pregnant (due to a higher risk of miscarriage) or nursing avoid or limit their consumption of foods, beverages, and drugs containing caffeine, for example OTC analgesics or decongestants. All sources of caffeine should be included when calculating your daily intake.

## Amphetamine/Methylphenidate Preparations

Other CNS stimulant drugs include the controlled substances (Schedule II) amphetamines (e.g., Adderall) and methylphenidate (Ritalin), which are used to treat attention-deficit hyperactivity disorder (ADHD) in children over age 6 years and for narcolepsy. Amphetamine/methylphenidate preparations are the first-line therapy for ADHD. Ritalin is also occasionally used in the treatment of senile apathy and major depression refractory to other therapies.

Daytrana is a transdermal system that contains methylphenidate in a multipolymeric adhesive matrix (making the drug difficult to extract) that is difficult to reapply once taken off. Vyvanse is a prodrug that is converted to dextroamphetamine in the GI tract and used to treat ADHD. Both products have the potential for a lower risk of abuse than other formulations.

The use of amphetamines to reduce appetite in the treatment of obesity is not recommended because tolerance develops rapidly and physical and/or psychological dependence may develop within a few weeks. *These drugs have a high potential for abuse and should be used only under medical supervision for diagnosed medical disorders.* However, when these drugs are used appropriately, as ordered by the physician, abuse potential (including other substances) and dependence appear to be minimal.

Side effects of the controlled CNS stimulants can include:

- Nervousness, insomnia, irritability, seizures, or psychosis from overdose
- Tachycardia, palpitations, hypertension, and cardiac arrhythmias
- Dizziness, headache, and blurred vision (dilated pupils with photophobia)
- Gastrointestinal (GI) disturbances, including anorexia, nausea, vomiting, abdominal pain, and dry mouth
- Habituation and dependence possible with prolonged use

An FDA review of reports of serious cardiovascular adverse events in patients taking usual doses of ADHD products revealed reports of sudden death in patients with underlying serious heart problems or defects and reports of stroke and heart attack in adults with certain risk factors. FDA recommends that children, adolescents, or adults who are being considered for treatment with ADHD drug products work with their physician or other health care professionals to develop a treatment plan that includes a careful health history and evaluation of current status, particularly for cardiovascular and psychiatric problems (including an assessment for a family history of such problems).

Precautions or contraindications for the CNS stimulants apply to:

Treatment for obesity (never more than three to six weeks) without diet and exercise modifications (weight gain resumes after discontinuation of the medication)

Anxiety or agitation

History of drug dependence, alcoholism, or eating disorders

Hyperthyroidism

Cardiovascular disorders

Closed-angle glaucoma (not modafinil)

Pregnant or nursing women

Abrupt withdrawal (depression results)

Use with monoamine oxidase inhibitors (MAOIs) (may cause hypertensive crisis)

Caution must be used with sustained-release preparations differing in designations (CD, ER, LA, SR) and their respective dosing requirements (see Table 20-1).

Pediatric precautions: Prolonged administration of CNS stimulants to children with ADHD has been reported to cause at least a temporary suppression of normal weight and/or height patterns in some patients, and therefore close monitoring is required. Growth rebound has been observed after discontinuation, and attainment of normal adult weight and height does not appear to be compromised. CNS stimulants, including amphetamines, have been reported to exacerbate motor and vocal tics and Tourette's disorder, and clinical evaluation for these disorders in children and their families should precede use of the drugs. Children should also be observed carefully for the development of tics while receiving these drugs.

There is some evidence that medication use only during school days may be tried in children with controlled ADHD, but only if no significant behavior or social difficulties are noted. Once controlled, dosage reduction or interruption ("drug holidays") may be possible during weekends, holidays, or vacations.

**Abuse of amphetamines:** Signs and symptoms of chronic amphetamine abuse and acute toxicity are discussed later in this chapter in the section entitled "Drug Abuse." Treatment of acute toxicity is also described in that section.

## Wakefulness-Promoting Agents

Modafinil (Provigil) is a psychostimulant medication approved for narcolepsy, sleep apnea, and shift-work sleep disorder in adults and adolescents (>16 years old). The potential for abuse and dependence appears to be lower than that for the amphetamines and methylphenidate. Modafinil is effective in treating ADHD in children and adolescents (but not adults) but was not approved by the FDA for this purpose due to serious side effects that developed with the doses used in clinical trials. It has also not been demonstrated to promote weight loss.

**Side effects** of modafinil (Provigil) for approved indications are infrequent and include:

> Mild headache, dizziness, nausea, and anorexia
>
> Anxiety, insomnia, depression, and mood changes
>
> Hypertension, palpitations, and tachyarrythmia

**Cautions** for the use of modafinil: Possible causes of fatigue and sleepiness should be determined before stimulant medicines are prescribed to increase wakefulness. Without adequate investigation, some common disorders, such as diabetes and sleep apnea, might go undiagnosed.

Reducing the necessary amount of restorative sleep for prolonged periods of time can result in mental and physical problems, especially neurological and cardiovascular effects.

# PATIENT EDUCATION

Patients receiving the controlled CNS stimulants should be warned regarding (utilize the Patient Medication Guide that is given out each time these products are dispensed):

> Potential side effects
>
> Potential for abuse and taking the medications only according to the physician's orders
>
> Taking the medication early in the day to reduce insomnia

The fact that abrupt withdrawal may result in depression, irritability, fatigue, agitation, and disturbed sleep

Watching for signs of tics, gastric disturbance, insomnia, weight loss, or nervousness in children receiving amphetamines and methylphenidate and reporting them to the physician

Potential for dangerous cardiovascular side effects

Not chewing or crushing sustained-release products

For parents and caregivers, the potential for abuse with stimulants and signs of abuse such as running out of the medication early, rapid weight loss, and unusual changes in behavior

Necessity for regular sleep in sufficient amounts to restore mental and physiological functioning to an optimal level while taking modafinil

# SELECTIVE NOREPINEPHRINE REUPTAKE INHIBITOR (SNRI) FOR ADHD

Atomoxetine (Strattera) is a selective norepinephrine reuptake inhibitor (SNRI) and the first *nonstimulant, noncontrolled* drug approved for the treatment of ADHD. Atomoxetine, structurally related to fluoxetine, does not have a potential for abuse, has less insomnia and less effect on growth, and has been shown to be safe and effective in adolescents and children more than 6 years old and adults with ADHD. It has a longer onset to therapeutic benefit and reduced efficacy compared to the stimulants.

Side effects of SNRIs include:

- Dry mouth, reduced appetite, and fatigue
- Nausea, vomiting, constipation, and dyspepsia
- Urinary hesitation or retention
- Increased risk of suicidal tendencies in children and adolescents ("black box" warning)

Precautions or contraindications for SNRIs apply to:

- Narrow-angle glaucoma
- Cerebrovascular, heart, or hepatic disease
- Possible growth disturbance during treatment

Interactions of SNRIs occur with:

- Methylphenidate (combination has not been studied)
- Beta-agonists, vasopressor agents, and quinidine
- Fluoxetine, paroxetine, venlafaxine, and MAOIs

See Table 20-1 for a summary of the CNS stimulants and nonstimulant medication for ADHD.

**TABLE 20-1** Central Nervous System Stimulant and Nonstimulant Medications

| GENERIC NAME | TRADE NAME | DOSAGE | COMMENTS |
|---|---|---|---|
| *Stimulants* | | | |
| caffeine citrate | Cafcit | PO 20–25 mg/kg one time and then 5–10 mg/kg per day | For neonatal apnea<br>*Caution:* Do *not* use caffeine and sodium benzoate |
| amphetamine mixtures | Adderall | PO 2.5–40 mg daily in one to three divided doses per day (4–6h apart) | For narcolepsy, ADHD (attention-deficit hyperactivity disorder) (>3 years old) |
| | Adderall XR | PO 5–30 mg daily | For ADHD (>6 years old) |
| lisdexamfetamine | Vyvanse | PO 30–70 mg q A.M. | For ADHD (>6 years old) |
| methylphenidate | Ritalin, Methylin | PO 2.5–20 mg two to three times per day ac | For narcolepsy, ADHD (>6 years old) |
| | Ritalin SR, Metadate ER | 10–60 mg divided doses (Note 8-h duration of action) | ER tabs, for ADHD, senile apathy, refractory depression |
| | Metadate CD, Ritalin LA | PO 20–60 mg q A.M.. | ER (extended-release) caps for once-daily treatment of ADHD |
| | Concerta | PO 18–72 mg q A.M. | Tablet shell is excreted intact |
| | Daytrana Patch | 10–30 mg daily to hip (Take 2h before needed effect) | Remove patch after 9h |
| modafinil | Provigil | PO 100–400 mg daily | For narcolepsy, sleep apnea, and shift-work sleep disorder (>16 years old) |
| *Nonstimulant* | | | |
| atomoxetine | Strattera | PO 10–50 mg one to two times per day | Only noncontrolled, nonstimulant for ADHD (>6 years old) |

# ANTIDEPRESSANTS

Major depressive disorder (MDD) is a mental disorder characterized by an all-encompassing low mood accompanied by low self-esteem and loss of interest or pleasure in normally enjoyable activities. MDD is a significant health problem that affects about 15 million American adults annually. A national survey indicated that more than 16% of Americans will experience MDD in their lifetime.

The exact cause of depression is unknown, but it may result from a chemical imbalance in the brain. Chemicals in the brain, like dopamine, serotonin, and norepinephrine, are known as neurotransmitters. Substances that travel across the synapse (contact point of two neurons) transmit messages between nerve cells.

If these neurotransmitters are reabsorbed by one nerve ending before they have had a chance to make contact with the next nerve cell, they cannot perform their function. In depression, there may be a shortage of the neurotransmitters dopamine, serotonin, or norepinephrine.

Antidepressant medications, sometimes called mood elevators, are used primarily to treat patients with various types of depression. The five categories in general use are the tricyclic antidepressants, the monamine oxidase inhibitors (MAOIs), the selective serotonin reuptake inhibitors (SSRIs), the selective norepinephrine reuptake inhibitors (SNRIs), and the heterocyclic antidepressants. Although symptoms may be relieved in the first month, it is generally advisable to counsel patients to continue antidepressant therapy for six to twelve months to prevent relapse.

The FDA has directed manufacturers of *all* antidepressants to include a "black box" warning that antidepressants increased the risk of suicidal thinking and behavior (particularly during the first few months of therapy) in short-term studies in children and adolescents with manic depressive disorder and other psychiatric disorders. There were no occurrences of suicides in any of these studies. Anyone considering the use of antidepressants in a child, adolescent, or young adult must balance this risk with the clinical need. Patients should be observed closely for behaviors associated with these drugs (e.g., anxiety, agitation, panic attacks, insomnia, irritability, hostility, impulsivity, severe restlessness, hypomania, and mania) and communicate the same with the prescribing health care provider.

## Tricyclics

Among the first antidepressants in clinical use, the mechanism of action of the tricyclics involves potentiation of norepinephrine and serotonin activity by blocking their reuptake. Their pharmacology also includes strong *anticholinergic* activity that is responsible for many of the side effects seen. Tricyclics may be lethal in overdose (cardiac conduction abnormalities or dysrhythmias).

The tricyclics have delayed action, elevating the mood and increasing alertness after two to four weeks. They are frequently given at bedtime because of a mild sedative effect. They should be used with caution (if at all) in older adults because of the strong sedative and anticholinergic properties of this drug class and the increased risk of falls. Tricyclics may be more effective than SSRIs in some cases of severe depression and are used as an adjunct in neuropathic pain control (see Chapter 19, "Analgesics, Sedatives, and Hypnotics").

Side effects of the tricyclics, such as imipramine (Tofranil), are anticholinergic in action and can include:

- Dryness of the mouth
- Increased appetite and weight gain
- Drowsiness and dizziness
- Blurred vision

- Constipation and urinary retention, especially with benign prostatic hyperplasia (BPH)

Sexual dysfunction

- Postural hypotension, cardiac arrhythmias, and palpitation

- Confusion, especially in older adults

**Precautions or contraindications** for tricyclics apply to:

Cardiac, renal, GI, and liver disorders

Older adults

Glaucoma

Obesity

Seizure disorder

Pregnancy and lactation

Concomitant use with MAOIs

SSRIs (increase tricyclic blood levels)

**Interactions** of tricyclics occur with:

Certain antiarrhythmics and some quinolones (QT prolongation)

Clonidine (causing hypertensive crisis)

CNS drugs and alcohol

# Monoamine Oxidase Inhibitors

The mechanism of antidepressant action of MAOIs involves increasing the concentrations of serotonin, norepinephrine, and dopamine in the neuronal synapse by inhibiting the MAO enzyme that degrades or breaks down these neurotransmitters.

The MAOIs, for example phenelzine (Nardil), are rarely used today because of potential serious side effects and numerous food, herbal, and drug interactions. They cannot be given until two weeks after tricyclics and other interacting drugs have been discontinued. These agents are typically reserved for refractory or atypical depression or those associated with panic disorders or phobias.

**Side effects** of MAO inhibitors are adrenergic in action and can include:

- Nervousness, agitation, and insomnia

- Headache

Stiff neck

- Hypertension or hypertensive crisis (can be fatal)

- Tachycardia, palpitation, and chest pain

Nausea, vomiting, and diarrhea

Blurred vision

**Precautions or contraindications** for MAOIs apply to:

Patients with cerebrovascular, heart, liver, and renal diseases

Children under 16 years

Pregnancy and lactation

Abrupt discontinuation

Interactions of the MAOIs with some drugs, foods, and herbal supplements can cause *hypertensive crisis,* manifested by severe headache, palpitation, sweating, chest pain, possible intracranial hemorrhage, and even death. Interactions may occur with:

Adrenergic drugs and levodopa

SSRIs and SNRIs (resulting in seizures, fever, hypertension, and confusion—"serotonin syndrome")

CNS depressants (resulting in circulatory collapse)

Foods containing tryamine, tryptamine, or tryptophan, such as yogurt, sour cream, all cheeses, liver (especially chicken), pickled herring, figs, raisins, bananas, pineapple, avocados, broad beans (Chinese pea pods), meat tenderizers, alcoholic beverages (especially red wine and beer), and all fermented or aged foods (e.g., corned beef, salami, and pepperoni)

Emsam (selegiline) is a selective MAOI (type B) administered as a transdermal patch indicated for the treatment of MDD in adults. Blockade of MAO enzyme reduces the metabolism of dopamine but not that of norepinephrine or serotonin. Transdermal administration allows for lower doses and direct absorption into the bloodstream, reducing the likelihood of a dietary tyramine–induced hypertensive crisis (see Chapter 22, "Anticonvulsants, Antiparkinsonian Drugs, and Agents for Alzheimer's Disease," for interactions and precautions or contraindications).

## Selective Serotonin Reuptake Inhibitors

SSRIs are considered to be the first-line medications for the treatment of depression. They are preferred because of fewer side effects, greater safety in cases of overdose, and increased patient compliance.

The antidepressants in this category selectively block the reabsorption of the neurotransmitter serotonin, thus helping to restore the brain's chemical balance. Drugs in this class include fluoxetine (Prozac) and sertraline (Zoloft). Therapy may be required for several months or longer. Symptomatic relief may require one to four weeks, and there is prolonged elimination of the drug. SSRIs do not significantly affect cognition in older adults. Fluoxetine and escitalopram (Lexapro) are the only antidepressants recommended for the treatment of MDD in adolescents (aged 12–17 years), and fluoxetine is also approved for children aged 8 years and older.

Side effects of the SSRIs may include:

Sexual dysfunction

Nausea and other GI effects (the most common side effects during the first two weeks of therapy, but often transient)

Anorexia and sweating

⊖ Insomnia, anxiety, nervousness, tremor, drowsiness, fatigue, dizziness, and headache

Bleeding (due to impaired platelet aggregation)

Hyponatremia (low sodium levels)

QT prolongation with citalopram (Celexa) doses >40 mg per day that can lead to abnormal heart rhythm, which can be fatal

Caution with SSRIs applies to patients with the following conditions:

Liver or renal impairment

*Suicide prone*

Diabetes

*Bipolar disorders* (may precipitate manic attacks)

Underweight

Eating disorders

Pregnancy and lactation

Abrupt discontinuation

Interactions of SSRIs are possible with:

MAOIs (never take concurrently)

Amphetamines, most antidepressants, certain analgesics (fentanyl, tramadol), antiemetics (metoclopramide), antimigraines ("triptans"), antibiotics (linezolid), and OTC products (dextromethorphan, St. John's wort, tryptophan) (can result in serotonin syndrome—a potentially life-threatening reaction to excessive serotonin activity in the CNS.)

Anticoagulants, antiplatelet drugs, NSAIDs, and aspirin (increased risk of bleeding complications)

## Selective Norepinephrine Reuptake Inhibitors

Duloxetine (Cymbalta) and venlafaxine (Effexor) are antidepressants that inhibit the reuptake of both serotonin and norepinephrine. They are also effective in patients with chronic pain (neuropathic pain, fibromyalgia, and musculoskeletal pain). Refer to Chapter 19 for details on these two agents.

Desvenlafaxine (Pristiq), also an SNRI, is the major metabolite of venlafaxine and is pharmacologically equiactive and equipotent to its parent compound. It is indicated for the treatment of MDD. The drug-related problems, warnings, and precautions associated with the use of desvenlafaxine are generally similar to those of other SNRIs.

## Heterocyclic Antidepressants

The second-generation heterocyclic antidepressants are comparable in efficacy to the first-generation tricyclic antidepressants but have differing effects on dopamine, norepinephrine, and serotonin and distinctly different adverse effect profiles. Bupropion (Wellbutrin) is considered an *activating antidepressant* (like most SSRIs) and can be useful in cases of severe depression characterized by extreme fatigue, lethargy, and psychomotor retardation. It is also useful in helping to reduce relapse rates in persons who are quitting smoking (see Zyban in Chapter 26) and those patients who experience sexual dysfunction with other antidepressants. Buproprion has a risk of seizures, which increases with higher doses.

Mirtazapine (Remeron) is a *calming antidepressant* that can be useful in treating agitated depression, mixed anxiety and depression, and fibromyalgia. A common side effect of mitrazapine is weight gain, which can be helpful in patients with a poor appetite. Trazodone is highly sedating and is used in low doses as a hypnotic. It can be useful in higher doses in older adult patients for treating agitation secondary to dementia and treating activation side effects caused by the SSRIs.

Side effects of heterocyclic antidepressants can include:

- Drowsiness—common (except bupropion)
- Insomnia, restlessness, agitation, and anxiety (with bupropion)
- Dry mouth, nausea, dizziness, and confusion
- Priapism or impotence (trazodone; discontinue the drug)
- Weight gain (mirtazapine, trazodone)

Interactions of heterocyclics occur with:

Other CNS depressants, including alcohol, may potentiate sedation (mirtazapine, trazodone) or increase the risk of seizures (bupropion).

MAOIs (never take concurrently)

Food may decrease incidence of light-headedness.

Caution with heterocyclics applies to:

Patients who are suicide prone

Patients with anorexia and bulimia (buproprion)

Seizure disorder

Cardiac or liver disorders

See Table 20-2 for a summary of the antidepressant agents.

# ANTIMANIC AGENTS

Bipolar disorder, sometimes called manic depression, is a mental illness that is characterized by severe fluctuations in mood extremes. Patients may experience high (mania) and low (depression) mood swings with a diminished capacity for daily functioning. The cause of bipolar disorder is most likely an imbalance in brain chemicals that affect mood. Without treatment, bipolar disorder is a debilitating condition that will not improve on its own.

**TABLE 20-2** Antidepressants

| GENERIC NAME | TRADE NAME | DOSAGE | COMMENTS |
|---|---|---|---|
| **Tricyclics** | | | |
| amitriptyline | (Elavil)[a] | PO 50–300 mg daily | All of these drugs interact with CNS drugs. Give at bedtime. |
| desipramine | Norpramin | PO 75–300 mg daily | Less sedation, anticholinergic S.E., and orthostatic hypotension |
| doxepin | (Sinequan)[a] | PO 50–300 mg daily | Also used topically for eczema (Prudoxin) |
| imipramine | Tofranil | PO 75–300 mg daily | Also effective for enuresis |
| nortriptyline | Pamelor | PO 25–150 mg daily | Older adults and adolescent patients need lower dose |
| **MAOIs** | | | |
| isocarboxazid | Marplan | PO 20–60 mg daily in divided doses | All of these drugs interact with many foods and other drugs, resulting in serious reactions |
| phenelzine | Nardil | PO 45–90 mg daily in divided doses | |
| tranylcypromine | Parnate | PO 60 mg daily in divided doses | |
| **SSRIs** | | | |
| citalopram | Celexa | PO 20–40 mg daily | Doses >40 mg associated with QT prolongation |
| escitalopram | Lexapro | PO 10–20 mg daily | May be better tolerated than Celexa |
| fluoxetine | Prozac | PO 10–80 mg daily | Delayed response, long half-life; take in A.M. |
| paroxetine | Paxil | PO 10–60 mg daily | Older adults 1/2 dose; take in A.M. |
| | Paxil CR | PO 12.5–62.5 mg daily | Do not give with antacids |
| sertraline | Zoloft | PO 25–200 mg daily | Take in A.M. |
| **SNRIs** | | | |
| desvenlafaxine | Pristiq | PO 50–400 mg daily | Do not chew or crush |
| duloxetine | Cymbalta | PO 40–60 mg daily | Also used for neuropathy |
| venlafaxine | (Effexor)[a] | PO 75–375 mg divided doses | Take PC to lessen nausea |
| | Effexor-XR | PO 37.5–225 mg daily | Do not chew or crush; swallow whole |
| **Heterocyclics** | | | |
| bupropion | Wellbutrin | PO 100–150 mg two to three times per day | Take early in the day; space doses at least 6h apart to minimize seizure risk |
| | Wellbutrin SR | PO 150–200 mg daily–two times per day | Space doses at least 8h apart |
| | Wellbutrin XL | PO 150–400 mg | Give once daily in the A.M. |
| mirtazapine | Remeron | PO 15–45 mg daily | Take at bedtime; sedation is common |
| trazodone | | PO 25–100 mg at bedtime for insomnia | Take pc to decrease dizziness and nausea; if drowsiness occurs, may give large portion of dose at bedtime |
| | | PO 150–600 mg in divided doses for depression | |

[a]This brand name is no longer marketed, but the name is still commonly used.

## Lithium

Lithium salts are approved for the treatment of mania and the treatment and prophylaxis of bipolar disorder. They prevent more manic episodes when compared with depressive episodes. Lithium is the only mood stabilizer that has lowered the suicide rate in bipolar patients. A maintenance dose is established by monitoring blood levels. Serum levels are checked seven days after starting or changing the lithium dose and every 6 to 12 months once a stable dose is established to maintain a level of 0.8–1.2 mEq/mL. Patients must be monitored and alerted for signs of toxicity.

Side effects of lithium can include:

- GI distress (usual initially and resolves—take medicine with meals)
- Cardiac arrhythmias and hypotension
- Thirst and polyuria (dehydration may cause acute toxicity)
- Weight gain
- Tremors (can be treated with propranolol)
- Thyroid problems—hypothyroidism, goiter

Signs of lithium toxicity can include:

- Drowsiness, confusion, blurred vision, and photophobia
- Tremors, muscle weakness, seizures, coma, and cardiovascular collapse

Caution with lithium when given to patients with the following conditions:

- Seizure disorders and parkinsonism
- Cardiovascular and kidney disorders
- Older adults and debilitated patients
- Thyroid disease

Interactions of lithium occur with CNS drugs, most antidepressants, diuretics, nonsteroidal anti-inflammatory drugs (NSAIDs), angiotensin-converting enzyme (ACE) inhibitors, and sodium salts.

The anticonvulsants valproate (Depakote, Depakene), lamotrigine (Lamictal), and carbamazepine (Tegretol) are also used for mood stabilization in bipolar illness (see Chapter 22, "Anticonvulsants, Antiparkinsonian Drugs, and Agents for Alzheimer's Disease," for details on these drugs).

Symbyax, a combination of the atypical antipsychotic olanzapine and the SSRI fluoxetine, is the first FDA-approved combination product for the depressive phase of bipolar disorder. In addition, the atypical antipsychotics aripiprazole, olanzapine, quetiapine, risperidone, and ziprasidone are approved to treat the manic phase of bipolar disorder. Refer to the discussion of these agents in this chapter for further details.

See Table 20-3 for a summary of antimanic agents.

**TABLE 20-3** Antimanic Agents

| GENERIC NAME | TRADE NAME | DOSAGE | COMMENTS |
|---|---|---|---|
| lithium | Lithobid | 900–1,800 mg divided doses | 0.8–1.2 mEq/mL (desired serum level) |
| carbamazepine | Tegretol, Tegretol XR | PO 600–1,600 mg in divided doses | 4–12 mcg/mL (desired serum level) |
| lamotrigine | Lamictal | Titrate up to PO 200 mg daily | May be more effective than lithium for preventing depressive episodes |
| valproate | Depakote DR, | PO 750–2,500 mg per day (divided doses) | 50–125 mcg/mL (desired serum level) |
| | Depakene | | IR capsule, liquid |
| | Depakote ER | PO 250–1,000 mg per day | For migraine prophylaxis |
| olanzapine/fluoxetine | Symbyax | PO q P.M. (various strengths) | For bipolar depression |

# ANXIOLYTICS

Anxiety disorders are present in over 13% of individuals in the United States. Anxiety is the body's natural response to real or perceived danger. This natural response becomes a disorder when it is excessive and difficult to control and when it leads to significant distress and impairment. Types of anxiety disorders include social anxiety, post-traumatic stress disorder, panic attacks, and obsessive compulsive behavior.

## Benzodiazepines

Benzodiazepines (BDZs) are sometimes referred to as anxiolytics or minor tranquilizers. They are useful for the short-term treatment of (1) anxiety disorders, (2) some psychosomatic disorders and insomnia, and (3) alcohol withdrawal. BDZs, such as diazepam (Valium), are also used as muscle relaxants, as anticonvulsants, in preprocedure testing, or preoperatively for sedation induction. Clonazepam (Klonopin), used primarily in the management of seizures (see Chapter 22), is also used in the treatment of panic disorder.

Anxiolytic BDZs, when given in small doses, can reduce anxiety and promote relaxation without causing sedation. Larger doses are sometimes prescribed at bedtime for their sedative effect. The role of BDZs in treating anxiety disorders is providing acute relief of anxiety symptoms while waiting for long-term treatment (e.g., SSRI or SNRI antidepressants) to take effect. BDZs do not treat the underlying cause of anxiety (abnormality of neurotransmitters) but rather only mask the symptoms.

Minor tranquilizers should not be taken for prolonged periods of time because *tolerance and physical and psychological dependence may develop.* Alprazolam (Xanax) is one of the most abused BDZs due to its quick onset of action, which leads to euphoria. All BDZs are classified as Schedule IV controlled substances. *Sudden withdrawal (missed doses/discontinuation) after prolonged use may result in seizures, agitation, psychosis, insomnia, and gastric distress.*

BDZs with a long half-life, such as clorazepate (Tranxene) and diazepam, should be avoided in older adults. Oxazepam (Serax) and lorazepam (Ativan) have medium to short half-lives and inactive metabolites and are less prone to accumulation in older adult patients or those with liver disease.

Side effects of the BDZs may include:

- Depression, hallucinations, confusion, agitation, bizarre behavior, and amnesia
- Drowsiness, lethargy, and headache
- Ataxia and tremor
- Increased risk of falls in older patients by ~50%
  Rash and itching
- Sensitivity to sunlight

Precautions or contraindications for BDZs apply to:

Mental depression

Suicidal tendencies; history of substance abuse

Depressed vital signs

Pulmonary disease and respiratory depression

Pregnancy and lactation

Children

Liver and kidney dysfunction

Older adults and debilitated patients (paradoxical reactions) and prolonged elimination time

Persons operating machinery

Interactions of BDZs with potentiation of effect may occur with:

CNS depressants (e.g., analgesics, anesthetics, sedative hypnotics, other muscle relaxants, antihistamines, and alcohol); NOTE: potentially lethal overdose when BDZs are mixed with alcohol or opioids

Antiretroviral protease inhibitors, macrolides (erythromycin), azole antifungals (ketoconazole, itraconazole), oral contraceptives, and calcium channel blockers (diltiazem, verapamil) all reduce the elimination of most BDZs, leading to increased and excessive sedation or impaired psychomotor function

Phenytoin (potentiation of phenytoin by raising serum concentration)

Grapefruit juice can potentiate the effects of orally administered alprazolam, midazolam, and diazepam, and should not be taken concurrently.

Midazolam (Versed) is a potent BDZ. It is used preoperatively to relieve anxiety and provide sedation, light anesthesia, and amnesia of operative events. Because of its more rapid onset of sedative effects and more pronounced amnesic effects during the first hour following administration, it is considered the drug of choice for short surgical procedures. Midazolam is usually administered IV, and the duration of amnesia is about 1h. It has also been used orally for preoperative sedation and to relieve anxiety with good results.

Midazolam may be used alone or in combination with an opioid such as fentanyl for painful procedures (e.g., endoscopy and cardiac catheterization with or without intervention). Midazolam is also used IV for the induction of general anesthesia, along with an opioid. This potent sedative requires individualized dosage with adjustment for age, weight, clinical condition, and procedure.

Side effects of midazolam can include:

⊘ *Depressed respiration* with large doses, especially in older adults and those with COPD (chronic obstructive pulmonary disease)

Paradoxical reactions (agitation or involuntary movements) occur occasionally

Nausea and vomiting occasionally

Cautions with midazolam:

Watch for apnea, hypoxia, and/or cardiac arrest

Respiratory status should be monitored continuously during parenteral use

Facilities and equipment for respiratory and cardiovascular support should be readily available; vital signs should be monitored carefully for changes in blood pressure or decrease in heart rate

Patients with electrolyte imbalance, renal impairment, and congestive heart failure and children are at increased risk of complications

Contraindicated in pregnancy and those with acute narrow-angle glaucoma

Interactions of midazolam, which can potentiate the possibility of respiratory depression, occur with:

Cimetidine (Tagamet) and ranitidine (Zantac)

Same medications listed under BDZs

## Other Anxiolytics

Other anxiolytics, not related to the BDZs, include buspirone (BuSpar) and hydroxyzine (Vistaril). Unlike the BDZs, buspirone has no anticonvulsant or muscle relaxant activity, does not substantially impair psychomotor function, and has little sedative effect. It is indicated for the treatment of generalized anxiety disorder but not other anxiety disorders; it does not have activity against depression. Limited evidence suggests that buspirone may be more effective for cognitive and interpersonal problems, including anger and hostility associated with anxiety, whereas the BDZs may be more effective for somatic symptoms of anxiety.

Buspirone has a slower onset of action than most anxiolytics (two to four weeks for optimum effect). Therefore, it is ineffective on a PRN basis. It has little potential for tolerance or dependence and has been used without unusual adverse effects or decreased efficiency for as long as a year.

Side effects of buspirone (fewer and less severe) may include:

Dizziness, drowsiness, and headache

GI effects (e.g., nausea)

Caution with buspirone applies to renal and hepatic impairment.

Another short-term anxiolytic, chemically different from the BDZs, is hydroxyzine (Vistaril). It is an antihistamine ($H_1$-blocker) structurally related to meclizine (Antivert). Hydroxyzine is also used IM as a pre- and postoperative antiemetic and sedative.

Side effects of hydroxyzine, generally anticholinergic in nature, may include:

Drowsiness, ataxia, and dizziness

Urinary retention and mydriasis

Caution with hydroxyzine applies to:

GI, hepatic, respiratory, and urinary disorders

Closed-angle glaucoma

Older adults

Pregnancy (especially first trimester)

See Table 20-4 for a summary of antianxiety medications.

### TABLE 20-4 Antianxiety Medications (Anxiolytics)

| GENERIC NAME | TRADE NAME | DOSAGE | COMMENTS |
|---|---|---|---|
| **Benzodiazepines (short-term use only)** | | | |
| alprazolam | Xanax | PO 0.125–0.5 mg BID–TID | Abrupt withdrawal may cause severe side effects; one of the most abused BDZs |
| | Xanax XR | PO 0.5–6 mg q A.M. | For panic disorder |
| chlordiazepoxide | (Librium)[a] | PO 5–25 mg TID or four times per day | Larger doses needed for ethanol withdrawal |
| clorazepate | Tranxene | PO 7.5–60 mg daily in divided doses | If used in older adult patients no more than 15 mg daily |
| diazepam | Valium | PO 2–10 mg TID, IV | Do not mix in syringe with other medications; also used as a muscle relaxant or IV in status epilepticus; R for refractory seizures |
| | Diastat | R 0.2 mg/kg | |
| lorazepam | Ativan | PO, IM, or IV 2–3 mg daily in divided doses | For older adults who are agitated |
| midazolam | (Versed)[a] | PO, IM, or IV dose varies with usage | Used preoperatively for short-term procedures |
| oxazepam | (Serax)[a] | PO 10–15 mg TID or four times per day | For older adults who are agitated |
| **Other Anxiolytics** | | | |
| buspirone | BuSpar | PO 15–60 mg daily in divided doses | Slow onset of action; may be used long term |
| hydroxyzine | Vistaril | PO 25–100 mg four times per day or 25–100 mg deep IM | Also used as an antiemetic and antipruritic or preoperatively |

[a]This brand name is no longer marketed, but the name is still commonly used.

# ANTIPSYCHOTIC MEDICATIONS/MAJOR TRANQUILIZERS

Antipsychotic medications, or major tranquilizers, are sometimes called neuroleptics and consist of the traditional or *typical* (first-generation) and the newer or *atypical* (second-generation) agents. They are useful in two major areas:

Relieving symptoms of psychoses, including delusion, hallucinations, agitation, and combativeness

Relieving nausea and vomiting, for example prochlorperazine (Compazine) (see Chapter 16)

Most of the typical antipsychotics in use today are classified chemically as phenothiazines; for example chlorpromazine (Thorazine) or butyrophenone derivatives such as haloperidol (Haldol). Dosage can be regulated to modify disturbed behavior and relieve severe anxiety in many cases without profound impairment of consciousness. These agents work primarily by blocking dopamine receptors, which accounts for their antiemetic effects but results in unbalanced cholinergic activity, which causes frequent extrapyramidal side effects (EPS) to include tardive dyskinesia (TD). The extrapyramidal system controls equilibrium and muscle tone, so EPS can include the muscle rigidity; tremors; difficulty walking; and involuntary, repetitive, and purposeless body movements called tardive dyskinesia. Despite their side effects, typical antipsychotics are still commonly used in the acute hospital setting because they are the only medications in this class available for IV administration.

The other class of antipsychotics, the atypical antipsychotics, for example risperidone, are chemically different from the phenothiazines, blocking both serotonin and transiently blocking dopamine receptors. This mechanism results in less potential for adverse effects, especially EPS and TD. The direct antagonism at the serotonin receptor (or the histamine-1 receptor), however, may account for the weight gain and other metabolic abnormalities seen with the atypical agents.

Although helpful in treating behavioral and psychological symptoms of dementia, typical or atypical antipsychotic drugs are *not* FDA-approved (black box warning) for the treatment of geriatric patients with dementia-related psychosis. Cerebrovascular adverse events (strokes, transient ischemic attacks, and cerebrovascular accidents), including fatalities (due to heart failure, sudden death, and infections), have been reported in older adults with dementia-related psychosis (Alzheimer's, vascular and mixed) being treated with antipsychotics.

Since there is no FDA-approved medication for the treatment of dementia-related psychosis, other management options (ruling out other causes, behavioral or environmental modifications, recreational activities, etc.) should be considered by health care providers. If antipsychotics must be utilized for dementia-related behaviors, they should be used at the lowest effective dose for the shortest duration necessary with appropriate documentation and justification of need.

Side effects of typical antipsychotics differ based upon the potency of the agent. Low-potency agents including chlorpromazine and thioridazine are more likely to produce sedation, hypotension, and anticholinergic effects.

The remaining typical high-potency agents, including haloperidol, fluphenazine, and trifluoroperazine, are more likely to produce EPS.

Side effects of all antipsychotics may include:

Postural hypotension, tachycardia, bradycardia, and vertigo

Anticholinergic effects (see Chapter 13 "Autonomic Nervous System Drugs"): dry mouth, constipation, urinary retention, blurred vision, fever, confusion, restlessness, agitation, and headache

Jaundice, rash, photosensitivity, or hypersensitivity reactions

Prolactin elevation with the typicals

Agranulocytosis with clozapine (can be fatal)

Metabolic effects (increased risk of hyperglycemia, insulin resistance, diabetes, weight gain, and elevated cholesterol) with the atypicals

Extrapyramidal side effects, severe CNS adverse effects, include:

Parkinsonian symptoms, for example tremors, drooling, dysphagia (more common in older adults)

TD (involuntary and maybe irreversible, abnormal orofacial movements such as tics—more common in older adults, especially females)

Dystonic reactions (spasms or abnormal muscle tone of the head, neck, or tongue—more frequent in children)

Akathisia (uncontrollable motor restlessness—more common in children)

Treatment of parkinsonian symptoms includes concomitant administration of an anticholinergic antiparkinsonian agent, for example Artane or Cogentin (see Chapter 22). *Prophylactic administration of these drugs will not prevent extrapyramidal symptoms. These drugs will not alleviate symptoms of TD and can make them worse.* Dystonic reactions usually appear early in the therapy and usually subside rapidly when the antipsychotic drug is discontinued. Trihexyphenidyl (Artane), benztropine (Cogentin), or diphenhydramine (Benadryl) are used to treat dystonic reactions.

Precautions or contraindications for antipsychotics apply to:

Seizure disorders

Parkinsonian syndrome

Cerebrovascular disease

Severe depression

Pregnancy

Blood dyscrasias

Older adults and children

Hepatic, cardiovascular, and renal diseases

Prostatic hyperplasia and diabetes

---

**NOTE**

Tardive dyskinesia may become permanent and irreversible, and no treatment has been shown to be uniformly effective. Therefore, the best treatment is prevention. Patients receiving antipsychotic medication should be assessed for TD at the start of treatment and at least every six months with the Abnormal Involuntary Movement Scale (AIMS) (see Figures 20-1 and 20-2) or Dyskinesia Identification System: Condensed User Scale (DISCUS) available from www.med-pass.com and other websites. Dosage should not be terminated abruptly in those receiving high doses for prolonged periods of time.

INSTRUCTIONS: Complete Examination Procedure (reverse side) before making ratings.

**Code: 0 = None, 1 = Minimal, may be extreme normal, 2 = Mild, 3 = Moderate, 4 = Severe**

| | | (CIRCLE ONE) |
|---|---|---|
| **FACIAL AND ORAL MOVEMENTS:** | **1. Muscles of Facial Expression**<br>e.g., movements of forehead, eyebrows, periorbital area, cheeks; include frowning, blinking, smiling, grimacing | 0  1  2  3  4 |
| | **2. Lips and Perioral Areas**<br>e.g., puckering, pouting, smacking | 0  1  2  3  4 |
| | **3. Jaw**<br>e.g., biting, clenching, mouth opening, lateral movement | 0  1  2  3  4 |
| | **4. Tongue**<br>Rate only increase in movement both in and out of mouth, NOT inability to sustain movement | 0  1  2  3  4 |
| **EXTREMITY MOVEMENTS:** | **5. Upper (arms, wrists, hands, fingers)**<br>Include choreic movements (i.e., rapid, objectively purposeless, irregular, spontaneous), athetoid movements (i.e., slow, irregular, complex, serpentine). Do NOT include tremor (i.e., repetitive, regular, rhythmic) | 0  1  2  3  4 |
| | **6. Lower (legs, knees, ankles, toes)**<br>e.g., lateral knee movement, foot tapping, heel dropping, foot squirming, inversion and eversion of foot | 0  1  2  3  4 |
| **TRUNK MOVEMENTS:** | **7. Neck, shoulder, hips**<br>e.g., rocking, twisting, squirming, pelvic gyrations | 0  1  2  3  4 |
| **GLOBAL JUDGEMENTS:** | **8. Severity of abnormal movements** | 0  1  2  3  4 |
| | **9. Incapacitation due to abnormal movements** | 0  1  2  3  4 |
| | **10. Patient's awareness of abnormal movements**<br>Rate only patient's report | No awareness 0<br>Aware, no distress 1<br>Aware, mild distress 2<br>Aware, moderate distress 3<br>Aware, severe distress 4<br><br>No = 0    Yes = 1 |
| **DENTAL STATUS:** | **11. Current problems with teeth and/or dentures** | No = 0    Yes = 1 |
| | **12. Does patient usually wear dentures?** | |

It is always preferable to perform the entire AIMS Examination. This establishes consistent testing conditions and allows test results to be compared. Nonambulatory residents may be observed informally for abnormal involuntary movements while in bed or in a wheelchair. Uncooperative residents should be observed during normal activities.

You must check one of these boxes: ☐ Full examination conducted and scored
☐ Scores from informal observations—Resident was:
☐ Not ambulatory—observed in   ☐ bed   ☐ wheelchair
☐ Not cooperative

| RATER | DATE: | PATIENT | Resident # |
|---|---|---|---|
| | | | |

**FIGURE 20-1** Abnormal Involuntary Movement Scale (AIMS). This test, or a comparable one, is performed every three to six months with all patients receiving antipsychotic medication to identify any signs of tardive dyskinesia.

## AIMS EXAMINATION PROCEDURE

Either before or after completing the examination procedure observe the patient unobtrusively, at rest (e.g., in waiting room).

The chair to be used in this examination should be a hard, firm one without arms.

1. Ask patient whether there is anything in his/her mouth (i.e., gum, candy, etc.) and if there is, to remove it.

2. Ask patient about the current condition of his/her teeth. Ask patient if he/she wears dentures. Do teeth or dentures bother patient now?

3. Ask patient whether he/she notices any movements in mouth, face, hands, or feet. If yes, ask to describe and to what extent they currently bother patient or interfere with his/her activities.

4. Have patient sit in chair with hands on knees, legs slightly apart, and feet flat on floor. (Look at entire body for movements while in this position.)

5. Ask patient to sit with hands hanging unsupported. If male, between legs, if female and wearing a dress, hanging over knees. (Observe hands and other body areas.)

6. Ask patient to open mouth. (Observe tongue at rest within mouth.) Do this twice.

7. Ask patient to protrude the tongue. (Observe abnormalities of tongue movement.)

♦ 8. Ask patient to tap thumb, with each finger, as rapidly as possible for 10–15 seconds; separately with right hand, then with left hand. (Observe facial and leg movements.)

9. Flex and extend patient's left and right arms (one at a time). (Note any rigidity and rate on DOTES.)

10. Ask patient to stand up. (Observe in profile. Observe all body areas again, hips included.)

♦ 11. Ask patient to extend both arms outstretched in front with palms down. (Observe trunk, legs, and mouth.)

♦ 12. Have patient walk a few paces, turn, and walk back to the chair. (Observe hands and gait.) Do this twice.

♦ Activated movement, some practitioners score these movements differently.

## INTERPRETATION OF THE AIMS SCORE

- Individuals with no single score exceeding 1 are at very low risk of having a movement disorder.

- A score of 2 in only one of the seven body areas is borderline and the patient should be monitored closely.

- A patient with score of 2 in two or more of the seven body areas should be referred for a complete neurological examination.

- A score of 3 or 4 in only one body area warrants referring the patient for a complete neurological examination.

**FIGURE 20-2** Abnormal Involuntary Movement Scale (AIMS). Examination procedure.

Interactions of the antipsychotics may include:

Potentiation with CNS depressants, anticholinergics, and antihypertensives

Drugs that prolong QT interval and increase the risk of life-threatening cardiac arrhythmias (antiarrhythmic agents, dolasetron, certain quinolones) with phenothiazines and ziprasidone

Dopamine antagonists (metoclopramide or promethazine), which increase the risk of TD and EPS

Antagonism with anticonvulsants (seizure activity may increase)

See Table 20-5 for a summary of the antipsychotic medications. See Figure 20-3 for a summary of the psychotropic drugs.

There is no "ideal" antipsychotic medication. Both conventional and atypical antipsychotic medications are associated with significant adverse drug reactions. However, research indicates a chemical component in many forms of mental illness. By altering abnormal levels of certain chemicals in the brain, such as serotonin, norepinephrine, or dopamine, many patients with mental or emotional illness have been helped. Psychiatric hospitalization has decreased since the advent of antipsychotic medications.

# PATIENT EDUCATION

Patients taking antipsychotic medications should be instructed regarding (utilize Patient Medication Guides where available):

The importance of being compliant with medication and nonmedication therapy

Potential for psychological and/or physical dependence with prolonged use

Caution in taking the medication only in prescribed dosage and for a limited period of time under medical supervision to reduce the possibility of serious side effects from overdose or prolonged use

Reporting adverse side effects to the physician at once (e.g., dizziness, blurred vision, nervousness, palpitations and other cardiac symptoms, urinary retention, GI symptoms, adverse mental changes, and EPS

Avoiding chemical abuse (e.g., alcohol, nicotine, or drugs) and obtaining professional treatment when these conditions exist

Possible severe withdrawal reactions (e.g., seizures) after prolonged use of psychotropic medications (withdrawal should never be abrupt, and medical supervision is indicated for prolonged administration of any of the psychotropic drugs)

Caution with interactions; *not* taking any other medications (except under close medical supervision) that can potentiate CNS depression (e.g., analgesics, *alcohol*, muscle relaxants, antihistamines, antiemetics, cardiac medications, or antihypertensives)

Not taking grapefruit juice with the BDZs, especially alprazolam and diazepam

*Older adult patients* are more at risk for the side effects mentioned earlier because of slowed metabolism and cardiovascular, kidney, liver, and visual impairment. They should be issued the following cautions:

Rise slowly because of the potential for hypotension.

Avoid operating machinery or driving while taking these drugs until you know how they affect you. Report to the physician immediately any side effects, especially dizziness, confusion, sleep disturbances, or weakness.

Avoid taking any OTC drugs or herbal supplements without medical supervision.

Tell the prescribing physician about all other medicines you are taking, including eyedrops.

**TABLE 20-5** Antipsychotic Medications/Major Tranquilizers

| GENERIC NAME | TRADE NAME | DOSAGE[a] | COMMENTS |
|---|---|---|---|
| **Typical** (*These drugs frequently cause EPS with long-term use. Monitor closely.*) | | | |
| ***Phenothiazines*** | | | |
| chlorpromazine | (Thorazine)[b] | PO 30–800 mg 1–4 doses daily, also deep IM, or IV | Primarily for agitation; also for nausea and vomiting and severe behavior problems |
| fluphenazine | (Prolixin)[b] | IM, PO 0.5–40 mg daily in divided doses | For older adults, reduce dose to ½ or ¼ |
| perphenazine | (Trilafon)[b] | PO 4–64 mg daily in divided doses | For psychosis, nausea, and vomiting in adults |
| prochlorperazine | (Compazine)[b] | PO, IM, or IV 5–10 mg | For agitation; primarily for nausea and vomiting in adults |
| | Compro | PR 25 mg BID | |
| thioridazine | (Mellaril)[b] | PO 50–800 mg daily divided two to four times per day | For psychoneurosis, agitation, or combativeness |
| trifluoperazine | (Stelazine)[b] | PO 1–20 mg BID | For schizophrenia and short-term for nonpsychotic disorders |
| ***Butyrophenone*** | | | |
| haloperidol | Haldol | PO, IV 0.5–30 mg daily divided two to three times | For agitation, especially with schizophrenia and delusions in older adults |
| | Haldol decanoate IM | IM 50–300 mg q4wk | |
| **Atypical** | | | |
| aripiprazole | Abilify | PO 2–30 mg daily  IM 9.75 mg (for agitation) | For schizophrenia; adjunct treatment for depression |
| | Abilify Maintena | 400 mg IM monthly | For schizophrenia maintenance |
| clozapine | Clozaril  Fazaclo ODT | PO 12.5–900 mg (divided doses) | Monitor WBC, neutrophil count; agranulocytosis risk |
| olanzapine | Zyprexa | PO 5–20 mg daily | Reduce dose by ½ for older adults |
| | Zyprexa Zydis | IM 10 mg (maximum dose 30 mg per day) | For acute agitation  Orally disintegrating tablet |
| paliperidone | Invega | PO 3–12 mg once daily | For schizophrenia; do not crush |
| | Invega Sustenna | IM 234 mg day 1, 156 mg in one week, and then 117 mg monthly | |
| quetiapine | Seroquel | PO 50–800 mg daily (divided doses) | Monitor for orthostatic hypotension |
| | Seroquel XR | | Also for depression associated with bipolar |
| risperidone | Risperdal | PO 1–4 mg BID | Reduce dose by ½ for older adults |
| | Risperdal Consta | IM 25–50 mg q2wk | For schizophrenia or adjunct therapy for bipolar disorder |
| ziprasidone | Geodon | PO 20–80 mg BID with food | Greater risk of cardiac disorders |
| | | IM 10–20 mg q2–4h (maximum dose 40 mg per day) | For acute psychosis/agitation |

[a] Varies with condition (divided doses).
[b] This brand name is no longer marketed, but the name is still commonly used.

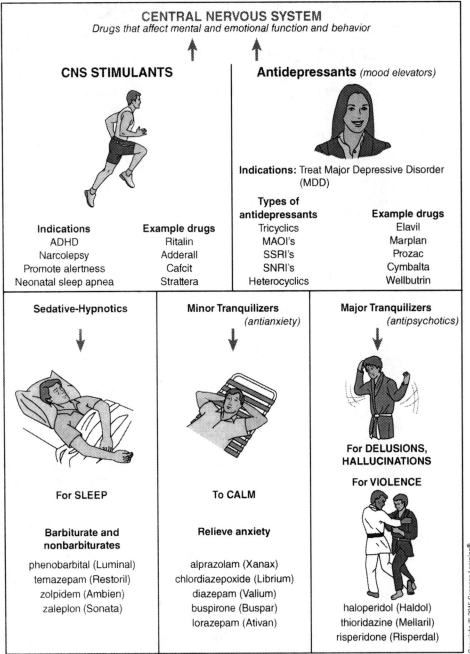

**FIGURE 20-3** Summary of psychotropic drugs.

# DRUG ABUSE

Drug abuse can be defined as the use of a drug for other than therapeutic purposes. According to the Substance Abuse and Mental Health Services Administration (SAMHSA), an estimated 22.5 million individuals in the United States are diagnosed with substance abuse or dependence. Of this number, an estimated 15.4 million people were dependent on or abused alcohol alone, 3.9 million were dependent on or abused illicit drugs alone (marijuana, pain relievers, and cocaine had the highest rate of abuse), and 3.2 million were dependent on or abused both alcohol and illicit drugs. A new report from SAMHSA stated that emergency department visits from the misuse and nonmedical use of ADHD stimulants more than doubled from 2005 to 2010, from 13,379 to 31,244; the greatest increase was among adults older than 18 years.

Drug addiction consists of the combination of all four of the following phenomena: tolerance, psychological dependence, physical dependence, and withdrawal syndrome with physiological effects. Habituation consists of psychological dependence only. Chemical dependency is the term used to describe a condition in which alcohol or drugs have taken control of an individual's life despite the problems related to their use and affect normal functioning.

# ALCOHOL

Alcohol (ethyl alcohol, ethanol) can be classified as a psychotropic drug and a CNS depressant. It is the number one drug problem in the United States, accounting for nearly 100,000 deaths per year, and is directly responsible for more than half of traffic accidents (one-third of all U.S. traffic fatalities). Alcohol is the most commonly abused drug among American teenagers.

Alcohol is a fast-acting depressant, pharmacologically similar to ether. The body reacts to alcohol with excitement, sedation, and finally anesthesia. Large amounts of alcohol can result in alcoholic stupor, cerebral edema, and depressed respiration.

Alcohol is rapidly absorbed from the GI tract into the bloodstream. Alcohol depresses primitive areas of the cortex first and then decreases control over judgment, memory, and other intellectual and emotional functioning. Within a few hours, motor areas are affected, producing unsteady gait, slurred speech, and incoordination. Prolonged use can cause permanent CNS damage and result in peripheral neuritis, convulsive disorders, Wernicke's syndrome, and Korsakoff's psychosis with mental deterioration, memory loss, and ataxia.

Prolonged alcohol use affects almost all organs of the body. Chronic drinking causes liver damage and pancreatitis. Alcohol irritates the mucosa of the digestive system, leading to gastritis, ulceration, and hemorrhage. Alcohol can also lead to malabsorption of nutrients and malnutrition.

Cardiovascular effects include peripheral vasodilation (producing the flushing and sweating seen with intoxication) and vasoconstriction of the coronary arteries. Alcohol increases the heart rate and, with chronic use, can cause cardiac myopathy, either directly or through metabolic and electrolyte imbalances. Potassium deficiency can cause cardiac arrhythmias.

Studies have shown an inverse association between the consumption of wine and coronary heart disease. In another study, it was determined that consumption of one or two drinks per day (five to six days each week) resulted in a reduced risk of myocardial infarction (MI) compared with nondrinkers. All this must be tempered with the deleterious effects of alcohol and the potential for abuse.

# Alcohol Poisoning

Symptoms of acute alcoholic poisoning include cold, clammy skin; stupor; slow, noisy respirations; and alcoholic breath. Mortality associated with acute alcohol poisoning alone is uncommon but can be an important factor when mixed with recreational drugs.

Treatment includes close observation for:

*Respiratory problems.* Establish and maintain airway.

*Vomiting.* Prevent aspirations.

*Seizures.* Do not require treatment unless status epilepticus occurs.

*Cerebral edema.* Diuretics sometimes required (e.g., mannitol).

*Electrolyte imbalance.* IV fluids with thiamine, folic acid, magnesium sulfate, and vitamins added ("banana bag").

*Alcohol withdrawal syndromes and delirium tremens.* Treated with IV BDZs.

Fetal alcohol syndrome (FAS) is a teratogenic effect of ethanol. As few as two drinks early in pregnancy has been associated with FAS, although it is more commonly seen in infants whose mothers consumed four or five drinks per day.

# Chronic Alcoholism

Symptoms of chronic alcoholism include:

Frequent falls and accidents

Blackouts and memory loss

Dulling of mental faculties

Neuritis and muscular weakness

Irritability

Tremors

Conjunctivitis

Gastroenteritis

Neglect of personal appearance and responsibilities

Treatment of chronic alcoholism can include an intensive in-house rehabilitation program in treatment facilities. Treatment frequently includes:

Vitamin B (thiamine) IV, IM, or PO; multiple vitamins; and folic acid

Low-carbohydrate and high-protein diet to combat hypoglycemia

Elimination of caffeine (in coffee, tea, chocolate, and soft drinks)

Reeducation of the patient, with intensive individual, group, and family counseling, including Alcoholics Anonymous techniques

### Pharmacologic therapy

Sometimes disulfiram (Antabuse) is used, with patient cooperation, as part of *behavior modification*. Patients receive daily doses of disulfiram and are taught to expect a very unpleasant reaction if even a small amount of alcohol is ingested. There is some evidence that drinking frequency is reduced but minimal evidence that it facilitates abstinence. This treatment is used less frequently because of severe reaction potential and poor compliance.

### Disulfiram—alcohol reactions can include:

Flushing and throbbing headache

Nausea and vomiting and metallic aftertaste

Sweating and dyspnea

Palpitation, tachycardia, and hypotension

Vertigo and blurred vision

Anxiety and confusion

## PATIENT EDUCATION

Patients taking disulfiram should be instructed regarding:

Not taking within 12h of alcohol-containing preparations

Avoiding cough syrups, sauces, vinegars, elixirs, and other preparations containing alcohol

Caution with external applications of liniments, lotions, aftershave, or perfume

Signs of disulfiram—alcohol reaction

Reporting to emergency facility if effects do not subside or with severe reaction

Carrying identification card noting therapy

Avoiding other medications that may interact with disulfiram (e.g., metronidazole, anticoagulants, and phenytoin)

Another treatment for alcoholism includes the use of daily maintenance doses of naltrexone (ReVia), as part of counseling programs, to keep alcoholics sober after detoxification. Naltrexone is a long-acting opiate antagonist, which acts by blocking the pleasurable sensations associated with alcohol (and opiates) and therefore lessens the desire or craving to drink. Naltrexone reduces the frequency and risk of heavy drinking but does not necessarily enhance abstinence. It is better tolerated than disulfiram.

### Side effects of naltrexone are usually minor and include:

GI side effects and decreased appetite

Headache, dizziness, and anxiety

Nausea and joint pains

Liver damage that can occur with doses larger than the recommended dose of 50 mg daily

CAUTION   If naltrexone is given to someone currently dependent on opiates, it can send the addict instantly into severe, life-threatening withdrawal. Initiate therapy only if opiate free for 7–10 days.

Precautions or contraindications for the use of naltrexone include:

Patients with acute or severe liver problems

# PRESCRIPTION DRUG ABUSE

According to the White House Office of National Drug Control Policy, prescription drug abuse is the nation's fastest growing drug problem. Prescription drugs are the second most abused category of drugs after marijuana, with nearly 22 million persons nationwide initiating the use of nonmedical pain relievers since 2002. According to the CDC, death rates from opioid overdoses have more than tripled since 1999 (in the United States in 2007, nearly 100 people died each day from a drug overdose).

Health care practitioners have ready access to many prescription drugs, and, therefore, sometimes become involved in the illegal misuse of controlled substances. Prescription drugs most often abused by medical personnel are hydrocodone, oxycodone, and the BDZs. Counteractive measures include accurate recordkeeping of all controlled substances and recognition of the side effects and symptoms associated with drug abuse. (See Chapter 19 for a discussion of narcotic analgesics and see discussion earlier in this chapter of the anxiolytics.) Report suspected abuse to the person in authority; follow specific state agency reporting requirements.

Treatment of opiate addiction (fentanyl, oxycodone, hydrocodone, etc.) consists of a combination of counseling, behavioral therapy, and medications. Methadone, naltrexone, and buprenorphine are the medications approved for the treatment of opiate addiction. Methadone (an opioid agonist discussed in Chapter 19), sublingual buprenorphine (Subutex, a partial opioid antagonist), and buprenorphine with the opiate receptor antagonist naloxone (Suboxone) can be used during the detoxification process and for maintenance treatment. Naltrexone (ReVia), a pure opioid antagonist discussed earlier, is used in the maintenance therapy to block the pleasurable effects of opiates.

# ILLEGAL DRUG ABUSE

This section describes four types of substances that can be produced illegally: the amphetamines, marijuana, cocaine, and the hallucinogens (LSD and PCP).

## Amphetamines

While amphetamines can be produced and prescribed legally, they are also produced in illegal labs. Two examples are methamphetamine ("crystal," "crank," "ice," "meth," "speed") and methylenedioxymethamphetamine (MDMA,

"Ecstasy"). At normal dosage levels, administration of an amphetamine may produce tolerance within a few weeks. However, in hypersensitive individuals, psychotic syndrome may occur within 36–48h of a single large dose of amphetamine. Some emotionally unstable individuals come to depend on the pleasant mental stimulation the drugs offer.

Symptoms of chronic abuse of amphetamines include:

- Emotional lability, irritability

  Anorexia

- Mental impairment, confusion, amnesia, and neurotoxicity

  Occupational deterioration and social withdrawal

  Continuous chewing or teeth grinding, resulting in trauma or ulcers of the tongue and lip

  Photophobia—frequently wearing sunglasses indoors

  Paranoid syndrome with hallucinations with prolonged use of high doses

  Tooth decay ("meth mouth")

Symptoms of acute toxicity from amphetamines can include:

- Strokes, cardiovascular symptoms including flushing or pallor, palpitation, tachypnea, tremor, extreme fluctuations of pulse and blood pressure, cardiac arrhythmias, chest pain, circulatory collapse

  Dilated pupils, diaphoresis, and hyperpyrexia

- Mental disturbances such as confusion, delirium, belligerence, combativeness, restlessness, paranoia, and suicidal or homicidal tendencies

- Fatigue and depression usually follow CNS stimulation

Treatment: There is no specific antidote for amphetamine overdosage. Treatment of an overdose is symptomatic and includes attention to airway, breathing, circulation, and administration of sedative drugs such as BDZs. General physiological supportive measures include treatment for shock or cardiac irregularities as appropriate. Administration of activated charcoal may help if it can be administered within 1 to 2 h after the substance was ingested. External cooling devices may be used to treat hyperthermia since antipyretics are not effective in this situation.

Abrupt withdrawal of amphetamines may unmask mental problems. Therefore, patients require careful supervision during withdrawal, and long-term follow-up may be required since some manifestations (e.g., depression) may persist for prolonged periods.

In an attempt to temper the meth epidemic, the Combat Methamphetamine Epidemic Act of 2005 (which took effect in 2006) banned OTC sales of ingredients commonly used to make methamphetamine. Pseudoephedrine (PSE), a popular and effective oral nasal decongestant, was the primary target of the act. PSE can now be stored and sold only under special conditions ("behind the counter") by pharmacies. Unfortunately, initial recordkeeping was store specific, and meth "smurfing" (the practice of going from one store to another in order to gain enough PSE to make meth) groups were formed to circumvent the law. In addition, Mexican drug cartels are filling the void with an inexpensive, highly addictive form of meth and sending it through the same pipeline already used to funnel marijuana and cocaine.

Chemically similar to methamphetamine as well as MDMA, the synthetic cathinones MDPV, mephedrone, and many others (collectively termed "bath salts") are an emerging family of highly addictive recreational drugs. "Bath salts" are designer stimulants not indicated for bathing but are falsely marketed as plant food, herbal incense, or more recently as jewelry or phone screen cleaner. The symptoms of abuse, toxicity, and treatment are similar to amphetamines, but the mental disturbances may be more prolonged, severe, and possibly permanent.

The DEA has classified MDPV, its salts, isomers, and salts of isomers as Schedule I substances (no accepted medical use) under the Controlled Substances Act. This regulation makes it illegal for anyone to sell or be in possession of these products. Unfortunately, chemists alter the chemical composition of the banned substance just enough that it still can be legally sold.

# Marijuana

Tetrahydrocannabinol (THC) is the active ingredient in marijuana. Although classified technically as a CNS depressant, it also possesses properties of a euphoriant, sedative, and hallucinogen. Marinol (dronabinol—a synthetic form of THC) is approved for the prevention of chemotherapy-induced nausea and vomiting and is also used as an appetite stimulant in cachexia associated with AIDS or cancer.

The *Cannabis* plant grows over the entire world, especially in tropical areas. Potency varies considerably from place to place and time to time. Its composition varies widely, and the methods of administration do not provide a standardized and reproducible dose. This makes it difficult to evaluate the potential therapeutic effects of marijuana for certain disorders, and it is illegal under federal law. Nevertheless, 18 states and the District of Columbia currently have legalized "medical" marijuana for (1) severe nausea and vomiting associated with cancer chemotherapy, (2) weight loss associated with debilitating illnesses, (3) spasticity secondary to neurologic diseases, (4) pain syndromes, and (5) glaucoma.

THC, the active ingredient released when marijuana is smoked, is fat soluble and is stored in many fat cells, especially in the brain and reproductive organs. THC metabolizes slowly. A week after a person smokes one marijuana cigarette, 30%–50% of the THC remains in the body, and four to six weeks are required to eliminate all of the THC.

Side effects of marijuana include:

- Short-term memory loss, impaired learning, and slowed intellectual performance
- Perceptual inaccuracies and impaired reflex reaction (dangerous with driving)

- Apathy, lethargy, and decreased motivation

  Increased heart rate, anxiety, and panic attacks

  Lung irritation, chronic cough, frequent respiratory infections

  Reduced testosterone level and sperm count

  Reduced estrogen level, crossing of placental barrier, and transmission through mother's milk; miscarriage and stillbirth possible

- Delayed development of coping mechanisms in children and adolescents

Another newer illicit drug class coming on the scene is the synthetic cannabinoids, known as "spice," "K2," "skunk," fake weed, and other names. These products, which are abused by smoking, contain dried, shredded plant material and chemical additives that are responsible for their hallucinogenic effects. Spice users report experiences similar to those produced by marijuana, but in some cases these are stronger with unpredictable effects (rapid heart rate, hypertension, seizures, acute kidney injury, and myocardial ischemia, and in a few cases spice has been associated with heart attacks).

Because the chemicals used in spice have a high potential for abuse and no medical benefit, the DEA has designated it as a Scheduled I controlled substance, making it illegal to sell, buy, or possess it. Just like the "bath salts" mentioned earlier, however, makers of spice products evade these legal restrictions by substituting different chemicals in their mixtures.

## Cocaine

Cocaine is a CNS stimulant and produces euphoria and increased expenditure of energy. The only approved medical use is as a local anesthetic, *applied topically only*, to mucous membranes of the laryngeal, nasal, and oral cavities.

Cocaine is highly addictive, causing dependence after even short-time use. It is abused by intranasal application (sniffing or snorting), intravenous injection, or inhalation (smoking "crack"). Nasal application can damage mucous membranes and/or the nasal septum. The effects of intravenous use are extremely rapid and dangerous and can be fatal. Smoking causes the most rapid addiction, sometimes after only one use. Cocaine crosses the placental barrier and has resulted in babies who are irritable, jittery, anorexic, and seizure prone. Cocaine use has caused numerous crimes and deaths. Severe depression can be associated with withdrawal, which is a lengthy and difficult process.

Side effects of cocaine, which are serious, include:

- Euphoria, agitation, and excitation
- Hypertension, chest pain, tachycardia, cardiac arrhythmias, or cardiac failure

  Anorexia, nausea, and vomiting
- Tremor and seizures
- Hallucinations, possible psychosis, and possible violent behavior
- Respiratory failure, strokes, and possible death from circulatory collapse

  Perforated nasal septum from prolonged nasal use

# Hallucinogens

Lysergic acid (LSD) and phencyclidine (PCP), an animal tranquilizer, are hallucinogens. They produce bizarre mental reactions and distortion of physical senses. Hallucinations and delusions are common with confused perceptions of time and space (e.g., the user can walk out of windows because of the impression that he or she can fly). PCP is also an amnesic.

Side effects of hallucinogens include:

- Increased pulse and heart rate and rise in blood pressure and temperature
- Possible "flashbacks" months later
- Panic or paranoia (lack of control)
- Possible psychotic episodes; chronic mental disorders
- Possible physical injury to self or others

# Dextromethorphan

Dextromethorphan (DXM), a semisynthetic morphine derivative, is a safe, effective, nonaddictive, OTC cough suppressant when used appropriately. Unfortunately, DXM (primarily the one found in Robitussin and Coricidin HBP products) is often abused by teens because of its phencyclidine-like euphoric effect, and the abuse of this agent may also be associated with psychosis and mania. The abuse of DXM can cause serious adverse events, such as brain damage, seizure, loss of consciousness, irregular heartbeat, and even death.

# Flunitrazepam (Rohypnol)

Flunitrazepam (Rohypnol), an illegal drug of a different type, is a potent BDZ that is approved for use in Central and South America for ethanol withdrawal. Not approved in the United States, it is being used here as a recreational drug (sometimes snorted to offset cocaine withdrawal) and is known on the street as "roofies." It has also acquired the title "date-rape drug" due to its ability to induce amnesia, preventing the victim from recalling specific events while under the influence of the drug.

# The Role of Medical Personnel

The role of the medical personnel in combating drug abuse includes:

Thorough knowledge of psychotropic drugs, action, and side effects

Willingness to participate in the education of the patient, the patient's family, and others in the community

Giving competent care to those under the influence of drugs in a nonjudgmental way

Recognizing drug abuse and making appropriate referrals without exception

Complete and accurate recordkeeping of controlled stocks of drugs that could be considered potential drugs of abuse

It is the responsibility of all medical personnel not only to recognize drug abuse but also to report any observed drug abuse to the proper person in authority. To look the other way not only enables the individual to continue to harm himself or herself but also endangers those in his or her care.

There are many services available to help medical personnel deal with drug abuse problems. Check with your state licensing agency or certification board for information about the programs in your area, such as the Impaired Nurse program. Local mental health clinics or psychiatric facilities can also provide assistance and information. Other agencies that can provide information include:

National Institute on Drug Abuse
www.nida.nih.gov
www.drugabuse.gov
www.clubdrugs.gov

National Institute on Alcohol Abuse and Alcoholism of the
National Institutes of Health
ww.niaaa.nih.gov

Substance Abuse & Mental Health Services Administration
www.samhsa.gov

Alcoholics Anonymous, Narcotics Anonymous
www.aa.org, www.na.org

# CASE STUDY A

## PSYCHOTROPIC DRUGS

Kevin McClellan is a 19-year-old college student who, by his roommate's accounts, has been displaying "odd" behavior. The roommate convinces Kevin to visit the student health center with him and reports to the nurse that Kevin has had periods of "wild activity" alternating with periods of lying in bed for days at a time. The nurse reviews Kevin's records and finds that he has a history of bipolar disorder.

1. What is the drug of choice to treat patients with bipolar disorder?
   a. Buspirone
   b. Chlorpromazine
   c. Alprazolam
   d. Lithium

2. Patients on lithium should be monitored for correct dosing by which method?
   a. Observation of patient's behavior
   b. Serum lithium levels
   c. Patient reporting of his or her own behavior
   d. EKG every three months

3. Side effects of lithium can include:
   a. Hypotension
   b. Hypertension
   c. Weight loss
   d. Hyperthyroidism

4. While reviewing Kevin's chart, the nurse notes that he has been visiting the health center during the prior school year with complaints of photophobia. This indicates which complication?
   a. Retinal detachment
   b. Potential seizure activity
   c. Lithium toxicity
   d. Dehydration

5. All patients should be cautioned when taking lithium with which category of medications?
   a. Anticholesterol
   b. Angiotensin (ACE) inhibitors
   c. Anticoagulants
   d. Sulfonylureas

# CASE STUDY B

## PSYCHOTROPIC DRUGS

Jose Aquilar is a 33-year-old marine who has just completed a six-month tour of duty in Afghanistan. He has been home for over four weeks and is experiencing signs of post-traumatic stress disorder.

1. Jose has asked his personal physician for a medication to help him cope as he assimilates back into his daily life. What type of drug would the physician be most likely to prescribe to Jose for short-term use?
   a. Antipsychotic
   b. Anxiolytic
   c. Tranquilizer
   d. Antimanic

2. The physician warns Jose that when taking a minor anxiolytic, he may develop drug dependence. What does this likely mean for Jose?
   a. He will need larger doses over time to achieve the same effect.
   b. He will associate the drug with incidents from his tour of duty.
   c. He will find it difficult to make it through the day without the drug.
   d. He will rely on the drug during any emotional conflict.

3. The physician also explains that sudden withdrawal after prolonged use of an anxiolytic may result in which symptom?
   a. Development of tics
   b. Somnolence
   c. Insomnia
   d. Blurred vision

4. Side effects of benzodiazepines may include:
   a. Akathisia
   b. Neuritis
   c. Dystonia
   d. Ataxia

5. Physicians should use extreme caution when prescribing a benzodiazepine to a patient with a history of:
   a. Kidney disease
   b. Substance abuse
   c. Type II diabetes
   d. Reflex sympathetic dystrophy

# CHAPTER REVIEW QUIZ

Match the medication in the first column with the classification in the second column. Classifications may be used more than once.

**Medication**

1. _____ Xanax
2. _____ lithium
3. _____ Risperdal
4. _____ amitriptyline
5. _____ Prozac
6. _____ Adderall
7. _____ BuSpar
8. _____ Zyprexa
9. _____ Ativan
10. _____ Wellbutrin

**Classification**

**a.** Antipsychotic
**b.** Anxiolytic
**c.** Antidepressant
**d.** CNS stimulant
**e.** Antimanic

**Choose the correct answer.**

11. Close monitoring of a pediatric patient taking a CNS stimulant for ADHD is necessary to assess for:
    **a.** Temporary suppression of growth pattern
    **b.** Alopecia
    **c.** Weight gain
    **d.** Hypotension

12. A side effect of a selective norepinephrine reuptake inhibitor (SNRI) for ADHD is:
    **a.** Growth retardation
    **b.** Insomnia
    **c.** Increased potential for abuse
    **d.** Increased risk of suicidal tendencies in children and adolescents

13. With depression, there may be a shortage of what substance in the brain?
    **a.** Glucose
    **b.** Dopamine
    **c.** Potassium
    **d.** Monamine oxidase

14. A common side effect of a tricyclic is:
    **a.** Weight loss
    **b.** Urinary frequency
    **c.** Mouth dryness
    **d.** Diarrhea

15. MAOIs can interact with some drugs and food and herbal supplements. These interactions can cause which side effect?
    **a.** Hypoglycemia
    **b.** Hypertensive crisis
    **c.** Seizures
    **d.** Hyponatremia

16. Tardive dyskinesia is characterized by which of the following?
    **a.** Muscle laxity
    **b.** Spasticity
    **c.** Tremors
    **d.** Involuntary, repetitive, and purposeless movements

17. Patients taking antipsychotic medications should be instructed:

    a. To take medications with grapefruit juice for better absorption
    b. To be aware that possible severe reactions may occur after short use
    c. To be aware that there is a potential for psychological or physical dependence with prolonged use
    d. To drink alcohol to calm the nerves if needed

18. A serious side effect of cocaine is:

    a. Paranoia                          c. Flashbacks
    b. Euphoria                          d. Panic attacks

19. The drug nicknamed the "date-rape drug," due to its ability to induce amnesia, is called:

    a. Rohypnol                          c. Fluticasone
    b. Lysergic acid                     d. Phencyclidine

20. Jared, a health care provider, suspects that another health care provider is abusing drugs. What is the first step that Jared should take?

    a. Give the individual the benefit of the doubt and remain quiet.
    b. Report any observed drug use to the proper person in authority.
    c. Confront the individual and threaten to tell a person in authority.
    d. Provide the individual with an 800 number for drug treatment and counseling.

---

**STUDY**GUIDE

**P R A C T I C E**

Complete Chapter 20

**Online Resources**LINK

• PowerPoint presentations

# CHAPTER 23

## ENDOCRINE SYSTEM DRUGS

## Objectives

*Upon completion of this chapter, the learner should be able to*

1. Identify the hormones secreted by these four endocrine glands: pituitary, adrenals, thyroid, and pancreas

2. Describe at least five conditions that can be treated with corticosteroids

3. Explain the administration practice important to corticosteroid therapy

4. List at least four serious potential side effects of long-term steroid therapy

5. Compare and contrast medications given for hypothyroidism and hyperthyroidism

6. Describe the side effects of thyroid and antithyroid agents

7. Identify the symptoms of hypoglycemia and hyperglycemia and appropriate interventions

8. Explain the uses and side effects of oral and injectable noninsulin antidiabetics

9. Compare and contrast insulins according to their action (rapid, intermediate, and long acting), naming the onset, peak, and duration of each category

10. Explain appropriate patient education for those receiving endocrine system drugs

11. Define the Key Terms and Concepts

## Key Terms and Concepts

Antidiabetic

Antithyroid

Corticosteroids

Endocrine

Hormones

Hyperglycemia

Hypoglycemia

Hypothyroidism

Immunosuppressant

Sulfonylureas

**E**ndocrine refers to an internal secretion (*hormone*) produced by a ductless gland that secretes directly into the bloodstream. Hormones are chemical messengers that have specialized functions in regulating the activities of specific cells or organs. Endocrine system drugs include natural hormones secreted by the ductless glands or synthetic substitutes. Hormones that affect the reproductive system are discussed in Chapter 24. This chapter covers four categories: pituitary hormones, adrenal corticosteroids, thyroid agents, and antidiabetic agents.

# PITUITARY HORMONES

The pituitary gland, located at the base of the brain, is called the master gland because it regulates the function of the other glands. It secretes several hormones such as somatotropin, adrenocorticotropic hormone (ACTH), thyroid-stimulating hormone (TSH), and gonadotropic hormones (FSH, LH, and LTH; see Chapter 24). The two pituitary hormones discussed in this chapter are somatotropin and ACTH.

The anterior pituitary lobe hormone, somatotropin, is called human growth hormone (HGH) because it regulates growth. Insufficient production of HGH will result in growth abnormalities, which should be treated only by an endocrinologist.

Adrenocorticotropic hormone (ACTH) is available only for parenteral use as corticotropin. Cosyntropin (Cortrosyn), a synthetic peptide of ACTH, is used mainly for the diagnosis of adrenocortical insufficiency. Treatment of associated disorders is usually reserved for the corticosteroids in which the dosage is more easily regulated and for which oral forms are available as well.

# ADRENAL CORTICOSTEROIDS

The adrenal glands, located adjacent to the kidneys, secrete hormones called corticosteroids, which act on the immune system to *suppress the body's response to infection or trauma.* They *relieve inflammation, reduce swelling,* and *suppress symptoms* in acute conditions. Corticosteroid use primarily can be subdivided into two broad categories: (1) as replacement therapy when secretions of the pituitary or adrenal glands are deficient (e.g., for Addison's disease) and (2) as anti-inflammatory and immunosuppressant agents.

Corticosteroid therapy is *not curative* but is used as *supportive therapy with other medications.* Some conditions treated with corticosteroids include:

*Allergic reactions* (e.g., to insect bites, poison plants, chemicals, or other medications) in which there are symptoms of rash, hives, or anaphylaxis

*Acute flare-ups of rheumatic or collagen disorders,* especially where only a few inflamed joints can be injected with corticosteroids to decrease crippling or in life-threatening situations, such as rheumatic carditis or lupus

*Acute flare-ups of severe skin conditions* that do not respond to conservative therapy; topical applications are preferable to systemic therapy, when possible, to minimize side effects

*Acute respiratory disorders* such as status asthmaticus (persistent and intractable asthma) (intravenous preparations are preferable) and sarcoidosis or to prevent hyaline membrane disease in premature infants by administering IM to the mother at least 24h before delivery

*Long-term* prevention of symptoms in severe persistent asthma or chronic management of COPD (oral inhalations are preferable for both conditions) at the lowest possible effective dose

*Malignancies* (e.g., leukemia, lymphoma, and Hodgkin's disease), in which corticosteroids (e.g., prednisone) are used with other antineoplastic drugs as part of the chemotherapy regimen; treatment of nausea and vomiting associated with chemotherapy (e.g., dexamethasone)

*Cerebral edema* associated with brain tumor or neurosurgery

*Organ transplant,* in which corticosteroids are used with other immuno-suppressive drugs to prevent the rejection of transplanted organs

*Life-threatening shock* due to adrenocortical insufficiency; treatment of other forms of shock is controversial

*Acute flare-ups* of ulcerative colitis; short-term use only to avoid hemorrhage

Prolonged administration of corticosteroids can cause suppression of the pituitary gland with adrenocortical atrophy, in which the body no longer produces its own hormone. To minimize this effect, intermediate-acting corticosteroids (predni-sone, methylprednisolone) can be given by alternate-day therapy when they are required for extended time periods. Withdrawal of corticosteroids following long-term therapy should always be gradual with step-down (i.e., tapering) dosage to allow the body's normal hormone production and regulation to return. Abrupt withdrawal can lead to acute adrenal insufficiency, shock, and even death.

Because of the potentially serious side effects, corticosteroids are administered for as short a time as possible and *locally if possible* to reduce systemic effects (e.g., in ointment, intra-articular injections, ophthalmic drops, and respiratory aerosol inhalants). Local administration reduces the dosage by avoiding the first-pass effect and going directly to the site of need. For *acute* episodes, some oral corticosteroids are available in *dose packs* (e.g., Medrol Dosepak, prednisone pak, DexPak TaperPak) to facilitate dose tapering.

Side effects of the corticosteroids used for longer than very brief periods can be quite serious and possibly include:

Adrenocortical insufficiency and adrenocortical atrophy

Delayed wound healing and *increased susceptibility to infection*

Fluid and electrolyte imbalance, possibly resulting in edema, potassium loss, hypertension, and heart failure

Muscle pain or weakness

Osteoporosis with fractures, especially in older women

Stunting of growth in children (premature closure of bone ends)

Increased intraocular pressure or cataracts

Cushing's syndrome, including obesity of the trunk, "moon face," acne, hirsutism (see Glossary), amenorrhea, and *hyperglycemia*

Nausea, vomiting, diarrhea, or constipation

*Gastric* or esophageal irritation, ulceration, or hemorrhage

CNS effects including headache, vertigo, insomnia, euphoria, psychosis, or anxiety

Petechiae, easy bruising, and skin thinning and tearing

Precautions or contraindications apply to:

Long-term use (regulated carefully; avoid abrupt discontinuation)

Viral or bacterial infections (used only in life-threatening situations along with appropriate anti-infectives)

Fungal infections (only if specific therapy is concurrent)

Hypothyroidism or cirrhosis (exaggerated response to corticosteroids)

Hypertension or heart failure

Patients with psychosis or emotional instability

Diabetes (drugs increase hyperglycemia)

Glaucoma (drugs may increase intraocular pressure)

Cataracts (cause or worsening of cataracts)

History of gastric or esophageal irritation (may precipitate ulcers)

Children (drugs may retard growth)

Pregnancy and lactation

History of thromboembolic disorders or seizures

Interactions may occur with:

Barbiturates, phenytoin (Dilantin), and rifampin (may reduce the effectiveness of corticosteroids)

Estrogen and oral contraceptives (may potentiate corticosteroids)

Nonsteroidal anti-inflammatory agents or salicylates (e.g., aspirin may increase the risk of GI ulceration)

Diuretics (potentiate potassium depletion, e.g., thiazides and furosemide)

Live-virus vaccines and toxoids (long-term or high-dose corticosteroids inhibit the antibody response)

Bupropion (dose-related risk of seizures)

Haloperidol (increased risk of QT prolongation)

See Table 23-1 for a summary of the pituitary and adrenal corticosteroids.

**TABLE 23-1** Pituitary and Adrenal Corticosteroid Drugs

| GENERIC NAME | TRADE NAME | DOSAGE |
|---|---|---|
| **Pituitary Drugs** | | |
| corticotropin (ACTH) | H. P. Acthar Gel | IM, subcu repository gel for injection |
| cosyntropin | Cortrosyn | IM and IV for adrenocortical insufficiency diagnosis |

*(continued)*

**TABLE 23-1** Pituitary and Adrenal Corticosteroid Drugs—(*continued*)

| GENERIC NAME | TRADE NAME | DOSAGE |
|---|---|---|
| **Adrenal Corticosteroids**[a] | | |
| cortisone | | PO for replacement |
| dexamethasone | (Decadron)[b] | PO, IV, IM |
| fludrocortisone | (Florinef)[b] | PO, for orthostatic hypotension |
| hydrocortisone | Cortef or Solu-Cortef | PO, IV, deep IM, subcu |
| methylprednisolone | Medrol, Depo-Medrol, or Solu-Medrol | PO, IV, deep IM, intra-articular |
| prednisone | | PO (tab or liquid); do not confuse with prednisolone |
| triamcinolone | Kenalog | IM, intra-articular (never IV) |

*Note:* Many other products are available. This is a representative list. Topical products are discussed in Chapter 12, and oral and nasal inhalation products are discussed in Chapter 26.

[a] Dosage varies greatly depending on the condition treated; large doses may be given for acute conditions on a short-term basis; long-term therapy can be given on an alternate-day basis with intermediate-acting agents, and dosage is reduced gradually to lowest possible effective dose.

[b] This brand name is no longer marketed, but the name is still commonly used.

# PATIENT EDUCATION

Patients taking corticosteroids should be instructed regarding:

Following exact dosage and administration orders (never taking longer than indicated and never stopping medicine abruptly)

Notifying the physician of any signs of infection or trauma *while taking corticosteroids or within 12 months after long-term therapy is discontinued* and similarly notifying the surgeon, dentist, or anesthesiologist if required

Taking oral corticosteroids during or immediately after meals or with milk to decrease gastric irritation

Taking single daily or alternate-day doses prior to 9 A.M. Take multiple doses at evenly spaced intervals throughout the day but not near bedtime

Avoiding any other drugs at the same time (including OTC drugs, e.g., aspirin) without the physician's approval (antacids or other antiulcer drugs are sometimes prescribed.)

Side effects to expect with the long-term therapy (e.g., fluid retention and edema)

Dangers of infection, delayed wound healing, osteoporosis, and mental disorders

Reporting any side effects to the physician immediately

# THYROID DISORDERS

An estimated 20 million Americans will develop a thyroid disorder during their lifetime. The thyroid is an endocrine gland located in the front part of the neck and is responsible for regulating the rate of metabolism. When thyroid levels are low, the pituitary gland releases TSH. TSH promotes the biosynthesis and secretion of the two bioactive thyroid hormones thyroxine (T4) and triiodothyronine (T3, the active form of thyroid hormone). Thyroxine is the major product of the thyroid gland, and much of it is later converted in the body to the active T3 form.

# Thyroid Agents

Thyroid agents can be natural (thyroid) or synthetic (e.g., Synthroid). Thyroid preparations are used in replacement therapy for hypothyroidism, the most common thyroid problem in the United States, which is caused by diminished or absent thyroid function. Synthetic agents, such as levothyroxine (Levoxyl), are generally preferred because T4 is a prohormone, and this allows the patient's own physiological mechanisms to control the production of T3.

Hypothyroid conditions requiring replacement therapy include *cretinism* (congenital; requires immediate treatment to prevent mental retardation) and *myxedema* or adult hypothyroidism due to simple goiter, Hashimoto's thyroiditis, pituitary disorders, medications (amiodarone, lithium), and thyroid destruction from surgery or radiation. Hypothyroidism causes slowed metabolism with symptoms ranging from fatigue, somnolence, dry skin, thinning hair, weight gain, constipation, sensitivity to cold, and irregular menses to mental deterioration (including depression) if untreated.

Transient hypothyroidism is rare, and thyroid replacement therapy for true hypothyroidism must be continued for life, although dosage adjustments may be required. Monitoring for toxic effects and periodic laboratory tests are recommended.

> **NOTE**
>
> The use of thyroid agents in weight reduction programs to increase metabolism when thyroid function is normal (euthyroid) is *contraindicated*, ineffective, and dangerous, leading to decrease in normal thyroid function and possibly life-threatening cardiac arrhythmias.

Toxic effects are the result of overdosage of thyroid and are manifested in the signs of *hyperthyroidism*:

Palpitations, chest pain, tachycardia, cardiac arrhythmias, and increased blood pressure

Nervousness, difficulty concentrating, tremor, muscle weakness, headache, and insomnia

Weight loss (in spite of increased appetite), diarrhea, and abdominal cramps

Intolerance to heat, fever, and excessive sweating; easy fatigability

Menstrual irregularities; exophthalmos (bulging eyes)

Precautions or contraindications for thyroid apply to:

Cardiovascular disease, including angina pectoris, myocardial infarction and hypertension

Older adults (may precipitate dormant cardiac pathology)

Adrenal insufficiency (corticosteroids are required first)

Diabetes (close monitoring of blood glucose is required)

Interactions of thyroid may occur with:

Food (can diminish absorption by 50%)

Potentiation of oral anticoagulant effects if added after warfarin therapy is stabilized

Insulin and oral hypoglycemics (dosage adjustment is necessary)

Potentiation of adrenergic effect (e.g., epinephrine; watch closely!)

Estrogens and oral contraceptives (decreased thyroid response)

Amiodarone (contains about 37% iodine by weight but can cause either hypo- or hyperthyroidism; monitor for changes in thyroid function)

Aluminum/calcium/iron/magnesium salts, chromium, and sucralfate (decreased absorption; space several hours apart if possible)

Soy products (decreased response)

## PATIENT EDUCATION

Patients being treated with thyroid medication should be instructed regarding:

Importance of taking the prescribed dosage of the thyroid medication consistently every day. It usually has to be taken for life. Take on empty stomach 30–60 min prior to breakfast

Importance of reporting any symptoms of overdose (e.g., palpitations, nervousness, excessive sweating, and unexplained weight loss)

Periodic laboratory tests to determine the effectiveness and proper dosage

Not changing from one brand to another or to a generic form without physician approval (if switched, TSH should be retested in six weeks)

## Antithyroid Agents

*Hyperthyroidism* can be caused by Graves' disease (an autoimmune disorder where antibodies mistakenly attack the thyroid gland) and thyroiditis (inflammation of the thyroid gland). Orally administered radioactive iodine ablation therapy is the most common treatment, and most patients are cured after a single dose. Surgery to remove all or part of the diseased thyroid is another permanent cure for hyperthyroidism but is seldom used now.

Antithyroid agents (e.g., methimazole or Tapazole and propylthiouracil or PTU) are used *to relieve the symptoms of hyperthyroidism* in preparation for surgical or radioactive iodine therapy or for those who are not candidates for either procedure. Methimazole is generally considered the treatment of choice because it works faster and is less likely to cause liver injury than PTU. Antithyroid drugs are not helpful for the treatment of hyperthyroidism associated with thyroiditis, since this condition is due to the release, not the overproduction, of thyroid hormones.

Side effects of antithyroid agents are rare and may include:

Rash, urticaria, and pruritus (treat with antihistamines)

Abnormal sense of taste

Blood dyscrasias (especially agranulocytosis)

Precautions or contraindications for antithyroid agents apply to:

Prolonged therapy (seldom used)

Patients older than 40 years old

Pregnancy and lactation

Hepatic disorders (black box warning with PTU)

Interactions occur with:

Other drugs causing agranulocytosis are potentiated

Excessive iodine intake or drugs containing iodine such as amiodarone (decreased efficacy)

## PATIENT EDUCATION

Patients being treated with antithyroid medication should be instructed to:

Take doses at regular intervals

Notify the physician immediately of signs of illness (e.g., chills, fever, rash, sore throat, malaise, and jaundice).

See Table 23-2 for a summary of thyroid and antithyroid agents.

**TABLE 23-2** Thyroid and Antithyroid Agents

| GENERIC NAME | TRADE NAME | DOSAGE |
|---|---|---|
| **Thyroid Agents** | | |
| levothyroxine (T4) | Synthroid, Levothroid, Levoxyl | PO, 25–200 mcg daily[a]<br>IV, 50% of PO dose initially |
| liothyronine (T3) | Cytomel | 5–25 mcg daily |
| thyroid (T3 & T4) | Armour Thyroid | 60–180 mg daily |
| **Antithyroid Agents** | | |
| methimazole | Tapazole | Tabs, 5–40 mg daily, in divided doses |
| propylthiouracil | PTU | Tabs, 100–400 mg daily in divided doses |

[a] When receiving orders for levothyroxine, caution is advised about decimal point placement (i.e., 0.025 mg vs. 0.25 mg) and dose conversions between mg and mcg, as medication errors have occurred.

# ANTIDIABETIC AGENTS

Diabetes mellitus (DM) makes up a group of hormonal diseases characterized by impaired metabolism of carbohydrates, fats, and proteins that results in elevated levels of blood glucose. Diabetes is fast becoming one of the most prevalent and costly diseases in America, affecting almost 10% of the population, with many people not even knowing that they have the disease or at the prediabetic stage. Prediabetes is a condition where blood glucose levels are higher than normal but not high enough to be called diabetes.

DM is classified as insulin-dependent Type 1 (characterized by the destruction of pancreatic beta cells) or Type 2 (characterized by insulin resistance and deficiency). Type 1 diabetes was formerly described as juvenile diabetes because it was usually diagnosed in children and young adults. However, adults can also develop Type 1 diabetes and require insulin. Type 2 diabetes is the most common (90%–95%) form of diabetes. There is an increase in children and young adults with Type 2 due to an increase in the rate of obesity at an earlier age.

The result of long-term, poorly controlled diabetes is vascular injury, which is categorized as microvascular or macrovascular. Common microvascular complications include retinopathy, nephropathy, and neuropathy. Common macrovascular complications of diabetes include coronary artery disease (including myocardial infarction), cerebrovascular disease (including stroke), and peripheral vascular disease. DM is considered to be the seventh leading cause of death in the United States; about 70% of diabetics die of heart disease or stroke. Health professionals of all disciplines have a responsibility to care for each patient in such a way that the risk of diabetic complications is minimized.

Medications that are administered to *lower blood glucose levels* include parenteral insulin and oral and injectable noninsulin antidiabetic agents.

## Insulin

Insulin is required as replacement therapy for Type 1 diabetics with insufficient production of insulin from the islets of Langerhans in the pancreas. Insulin is also required in patients with Type 2 diabetes who have failed to maintain satisfactory concentrations of blood glucose with therapy including dietary regulation and oral antidiabetic agents. Insulin is also indicated for stable Type 2 diabetics at the time of surgery, fever, severe trauma, infection, serious renal or hepatic dysfunction, endocrine dysfunction, gangrene, or pregnancy. Insulin (regular) is used in the emergency treatment of diabetic ketoacidosis or coma.

Insulin must be administered parenterally because it is destroyed in the GI tract. All *injected* insulin products currently marketed are one of two types: biosynthetic human or analog. Biosynthetic insulins are referred to as "human" because their amino acid structure is identical to naturally occurring human insulin. Analog insulin (aspart, detemir, glargine, glulisine, and lispro) differs from human insulin only by substitution or position changes in the human insulin molecule, which mimics normal insulin secretion better than traditional insulins and reduces hypoglycemia. Biosynthetic and analog insulins are created using recombinant DNA technology.

Most of the insulin used today is U-100, which means that there are 100 units of insulin in each milliliter. The insulin syringe *must be marked U-100* to match the insulin used. Remember that on the 100 unit (1 mL) insulin syringe each line represents two units. If a smaller 50 unit (1/2 mL) syringe is used, each line represents one unit of insulin (see Chapters 4 and 9 for details). *Always have a clinician compare the insulin in the syringe with the dosage ordered to prevent errors,* which could have serious consequences. Another delivery option is prefilled insulin pens, which offer convenience and may help to avoid certain types of medication errors. In addition, implantable programmable insulin pumps are available that can administer insulin continuously through a catheter. Some pumps have internal glucose sensors to monitor levels. See Figure 23-1.

Insulin preparations differ mainly in their onset, peak, and duration of action (Table 23-3). Aspart, glulisine, and lispro insulins are ultra-*rapid acting* and have a *very short duration* of action. *Regular* insulin is *rapid acting* and has a *short duration. Regular* insulin may be given intravenously and intramuscularly as well as subcutaneously. Aspart, glulisine, and lispro are clear and rapid acting (onset in approximately 15 min). They peak in about 1h and last approximately 4h. They may be given subcutaneously or intravenously. *Isophane* (NPH) is intermediate acting; glargine and detemir are long acting, and they are administered subcutaneously.

*Rapid- or short-acting* insulin is sometimes combined with isophane insulin in the same syringe. When two insulins are ordered at the same time, the *rapid- or short-acting insulin should be drawn into the syringe first.* Combinations of NPH and regular insulin are also available, for example Humulin 70/30 or Novolin 70/30. This combination provides rapid onset with a duration of up to 24h. Insulin *glargine* and insulin mixtures should not be mixed with any of the other available types of insulin.

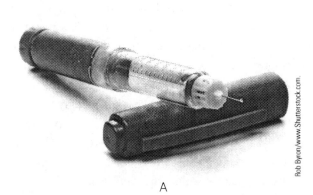
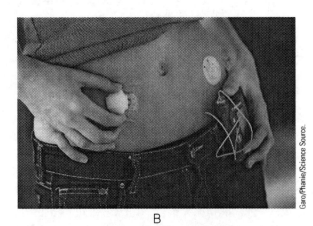

A                                                    B

**FIGURE 23-1** (A) Insulin pen: adjustable insulin dosage pen to regulate blood sugar levels. (B) Insulin pump: programmable implanted insulin pump administering continuous insulin subcutaneously to the fatty tissue layer. This pump has a glucose sensor to monitor glucose levels and adjust dosages.

| TABLE 23-3 Insulins | | | | | |
| --- | --- | --- | --- | --- | --- |
| **ACTION** | **PREPARATION** | **TRADE NAME** | **ONSET** | **PEAK** | **DURATION** |
| Rapid | aspart | Novolog | 10–30 min | 1–2 h | 3–8 h |
| | glulisine | Apidra | | | |
| | lispro | Humalog | | | |
| Short | regular | Humulin R | 30–60 min | 1–5 h | 6–10 h |
| | | Novolin R | | | |
| Intermediate | isophane (NPH) | Humulin N | 1–3 h | 6–12 h | 18–24 h |
| | | Novolin N | | | |
| Long | glargine | Lantus | 1–2 h | No pronounced peak | up to 24 h (dose dependent) |
| | detemir | Levemir | | | |
| Mixtures | NPH/reg | Humulin/Novolin 70/30, 50/50 | 30–60 min | 1–4 h | 16–24 h |
| | NPH/lispro | Humalog Mix 75/25, 50/50 | 15–30 min | 1–6 h | 12–24 h |
| | NPH/aspart | Novolog Mix 70/30 | 10–20 min | 1–4 h | up to 24 h |

**Note:** This is a representative list. Other insulin products are also available. Dosage varies. Due to limited use, beef- and pork-derived insulins and lente and ultralente insulins are no longer available in the United States. Before giving insulin, always check the expiration date on the vial and be sure that regular, aspart, glulisine, and lispro insulins are clear and isophane insulins are cloudy. Isophane insulins are administered only subcutaneously, never IV. Rotate administration sites with each injection. Levemir, Novolin N, R, and 70/30 can be used for up to 42 days after opening when stored at room temperature. Opened vials of all other types of insulin may be stored at room temperature without loss of potency for 28 days. Stability of insulin pens and cartridges at room temperature vary depending on the product; they are never to be shared among patients as this may result in the transmission of blood-borne pathogens.

Diabetes therapy with insulin focuses initially on controlling fasting plasma glucose with the use of a long-acting insulin analog (Lantus or Levemir). If further glycemic control is needed, a mealtime (also known as bolus or prandial) rapid- or short-acting insulin may be added to reduce postmeal hyperglycemia. Regular insulin is best given 30–60 min before a meal. The rapid-acting insulins can generally be given 15 min before or immediately after a meal. Insulin mixtures should be given within 15 min before a meal.

*Rapid- or short-acting* insulin is sometimes ordered as *corrective dose insulin.* This means that the blood is tested for glucose and a specific amount of the insulin is administered subcutaneously based on the glucose level shown by the test. Doses are adjusted according to blood glucose response and insulin resistance (the amount of daily insulin required by patients in low-, medium-, and high-dose categories). For example, the physician might write an order to give rapid- or short-acting insulin subcutaneously with the following corrective dose scale according to the blood glucose levels:

| Blood Glucose | Dosage of Rapid- or Short-acting Insulin | | |
|---|---|---|---|
| | **Low** | **Medium** | **High** |
| >350 | 5 units | 8 units | 12 units & Call physician |
| 301–350 | 4 units | 7 units | 10 units |
| 251–300 | 3 units | 5 units | 7 units |
| 201–250 | 2 units | 3 units | 4 units |
| 151–200 | 1 unit | 2 units | 3 units |
| 120–150 | 0 unit | 1 unit | 2 units |
| <120 | No insulin | | |

Remember, this is only a *sample* corrective dose scale. It is now recommended that the traditional sliding scale coverage be reserved for patients who are newly diagnosed as diabetic to establish insulin requirements, started on enteral or parenteral nutrition, or started on glucocorticoids (e.g., prednisone). *Always check the physician's order carefully to determine the exact dosage of insulin, which varies with the individual.* Verification of insulin dosage with another caregiver is very important to prevent one of the most common and most dangerous of medication errors.

There are many different types of insulins available, and many have names or packages that look or sound alike. There has been confusion between "Lente" and "Lantus" and "Humulin" and "Humalog." Confusion is also possible with the premixed products "Humulin 70/30," "Humalog Mix 75/25," "Novolog Mix 70/30," and "Novolin 70/30." *Be extremely careful to give the right insulin and the right dose! If in doubt, consult the pharmacist.*

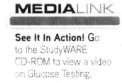

**MEDIA**LINK

**See It In Action!** Go to the StudyWARE CD-ROM to view a video on Glucose Testing.

# Hyperglycemia

Hyperglycemia, or elevated blood glucose, may result from:

Undiagnosed diabetes

Insufficient insulin dose

Infections

Surgical or other trauma

Emotional stress

Other endocrine disorders

Medications (e.g., glucocorticoids such as prednisone)

Pregnancy

Symptoms of hyperglycemia may include:

Dehydration and excessive thirst

Anorexia and unexplained weight loss in persons under 40 years old

Polyuria (frequent urination)

Fruity breath

Lethargy, weakness, flu symptoms, and coma if untreated

Vision problems

Ketoacidosis (can be determined by testing urine for acetone)

Treatment of acute hyperglycemia includes:

IV fluids to correct electrolyte imbalance

Adding *regular* insulin to IV fluids

Interactions: Insulin action is antagonized by corticosteroids or epinephrine, necessitating increased insulin dosage. Atypical antipsychotics, protease inhibitors, thiazide diuretics, oral contraceptives, and estrogen may also increase insulin requirements. Beta-blockers (nonselective) with insulin pose risks of hypoglycemia or hyperglycemia and can mask the signs and symptoms (especially tachycardia) of hypoglycemia. Thiazolidinediones (Actos and Avandia) with insulin result in an increased risk of heart failure and edema.

Interactions of insulin with *potentiation of hypoglycemic effect* occur with:

Alcohol

Monoamine oxidase inhibitors (MAOIs)

Salicylates

Anabolic steroids

## Hypoglycemia

It is estimated that 90% of all patients receiving insulin will experience a hypoglycemic event. Hypoglycemia, or lowered blood glucose, may result from:

Overdose of insulin and/or other antidiabetic medications

Delayed or insufficient food intake (e.g., dieting)

Excessive or unusual exercise

Change in the type of insulin, for example, from analog to human insulin

Symptoms of hypoglycemia may develop suddenly and are manifested usually at the peak of insulin action, including:

Increased perspiration, pallor, hunger, nausea, and vomiting

Irritability, confusion, or sudden unexplained bizarre moodiness or behavior change

Tremor, weakness, headache, hypothermia, or tingling of the fingers

Blurred or double vision

Tachycardia and shallow breathing

Loss of consciousness and convulsions if untreated

Hypoglycemic reactions in older diabetics may mimic a CVA (cerebrovascular accident)

Treatment of hypoglycemia includes:

> If conscious, administration of 4 oz orange juice, candy, honey, or syrup (especially sublingual for faster absorption). After initial treatment, provide a protein snack, for example peanut butter, cheese, or a glass of milk. Then recheck blood glucose.

> If comatose, administration of 10–30 mL of 50% dextrose solution IV or administration of 0.5–1 unit of glucagon (1 mg) SC, IM, or IV—follow with carbohydrate snack when the patient awakens to prevent secondary hypoglycemia.

> Avoid giving excessive amounts of sugar or frequent overdoses of insulin, which can result in rebound hyperglycemia (Somogyi effect) from an accelerated release of glucagon. Treatment of rebound hyperglycemia involves reduction of insulin dosage with continuous monitoring of blood glucose.

## Oral and Injectable Noninsulin Antidiabetic Agents

Type 2 diabetes results from insulin resistance (insulin produced but not used effectively by cells) combined with relative insulin deficiency. Type 2 diabetes is the leading cause of kidney failure, lower-limb amputations, and new cases of adult blindness. Patients may sometimes be treated with diet alone, that is, a low-calorie, low-fat diet; avoiding simple sugars and alcohol; and substituting complex carbohydrates, such as whole-grain bread and cereals, brown rice, and vegetables high in fiber.

Frequently, however, it is necessary to combine diet and oral antidiabetic agents. Oral antidiabetic agents may be administered as a single daily dose before breakfast or two divided doses daily, before morning and evening meals. These medications are not a substitute for dietary management. Weight reduction, exercise, education, and modified diet are still considered the principal therapy for the management of Type 2 diabetes.

Symptoms of Type 2 diabetes may include:

> Excessive weight gain after age 40

> Excessive thirst (polydipsia)

> Excessive urination (polyuria)

> Excessive weakness, poor circulation, and slow healing

> Visual problems

Oral and injectable noninsulin antidiabetic agents are available in several pharmacological classes with differing mechanisms of action, offering different avenues for reducing glucose levels. Because they work at different sites, they are often synergistic; some may be used in combination with one another or with insulin.

# Sulfonylureas

The oral hypoglycemic drugs known as sulfonylureas consist of first-generation agents (e.g., chlorpropamide, tolbutamide) and second-generation agents (e.g., glipizide, glyburide). The second-generation agents have mostly replaced the first-generation agents because of higher potency, shorter duration of action, better tolerance, and fewer drug interactions. The sulfonylureas work by increasing insulin production from the pancreas and by improving peripheral insulin activity. Although patients initially respond well to this class of drugs, glycemic control begins to wane after one to two years in most patients.

Side effects of sulfonylureas may include:

- GI distress (may subside with dosage regulation)

    Dermatological effects, including pruritus, rash, urticaria, or photosensitivity

    Hepatic dysfunction, including jaundice (rare)

- Weakness, fatigue, lethargy, vertigo, and headache

    Blood dyscrasias, including anemia

- Hypoglycemia, especially in older adults

    Possible increased risk of cardiovascular death (controversial)

    Weight gain and water retention

Precautions or contraindications for sulfonylureas apply to:

Debilitated or malnourished patients

Impaired liver and kidney function

Unstable diabetes or Type 1 diabetes

Major surgery, severe infection, and severe trauma

Older adults (refer to Beers List in Chapter 27; chlorpropamide and glyburide, which have a longer half-life, greater chance of hypoglycemia, and also a risk of inappropriate antidiuretic hormone secretion [water intoxication])

Interactions of sulfonylureas with *potentiation* of hypoglycemic effect can occur with:

Beta-blockers, MAOIs, or probenecid

Alcohol with facial flushing (disulfiram-like reaction)

Cimetidine, miconazole, fluconazole, quinolones, or sulfonamides

Salicylates and other nonsteroidal anti-inflammatory drugs (NSAIDs)

Interactions *with antagonistic action* (larger dose may be required) can occur with:

Thyroid hormones

Thiazide and nonthiazide diuretics

> Corticosteroids and phenothiazines
>
> Estrogens and oral contraceptives
>
> Calcium channel blockers
>
> Rifampin and isoniazid

When these agents are administered or discontinued in patients receiving sulfonylureas, the patient should be observed closely for loss of diabetic control.

## Alpha-Glucosidase Inhibitors

Alpha-glucosidase inhibitors such as acarbose (Precose) delay digestion of complex carbohydrates (e.g., starch) and subsequent absorption of glucose, resulting in a smaller rise in blood glucose concentrations following meals. Acarbose can be used as monotherapy or part of a combination regimen that includes insulin, metformin, or an oral sulfonylurea.

Side effects of alpha-glucosidase inhibitors may include:

> ❗ High rate of GI effects (flatulence, abdominal distention/pain, loose stools), which tend to diminish with time or a reduction in dose; take at the start (with the first bite) of main meals
>
> Elevated liver enzymes (dose-related, generally asymptomatic, and reversible)

Precautions or contraindications for alpha-glucosidase inhibitors apply to:

> Impaired liver and kidney function
>
> Patients with inflammatory bowel disease or intestinal obstruction
>
> Pregnancy and lactation
>
> Children

Drug interactions occur between alpha-glucosidase inhibitors and:

> Digestive enzymes (effect of acarbose reduced)
>
> Digoxin (reduced serum digoxin concentrations)
>
> Estrogens and oral contraceptives (impaired glucose tolerance)

## Biguanides

The biguanides, for example metformin (Glucophage), work by decreasing hepatic glucose production and enhancing insulin uptake in muscle tissue. Metformin is the preferred initial first-line monotherapy or can be used in combination with sulfonylureas, alpha-glucosidase inhibitors, or insulin to treat Type 2 diabetics.

Side effects of biguanides may include:

> ❗ GI effects (diarrhea, nausea, vomiting, bloating, flatulence, metallic taste, anorexia, and weight loss), which are generally mild and resolve

during treatment; can take the medication with food to minimize epigastric discomfort

Lactic acidosis (a rare but serious metabolic complication) in patients with a history of ketoacidosis, severe dehydration, cardiorespiratory insufficiency, renal dysfunction, and chronic alcoholism with liver damage

Vitamin $B_{12}$ deficiency (patients may present with peripheral neuropathy)

Hypoglycemia (rare when used without sulfonylureas or insulin)

**Precautions or contraindications** for biguanides apply to:

Impaired liver and kidney function

Patients with heart failure requiring pharmacologic treatment

Administration of radiocontrast dye (could result in acute alteration of renal function; withhold metformin just prior to tests with radioactive dye and for 48h after completion of the procedure)

Pregnancy and lactation

Children and older adults (especially those who are frail, anorexic, or underweight)

**Drug interactions** with biguanides include:

Increased metformin effect seen with alcohol, cephalexin, and cimetidine

Radiopaque contrast media (see contraindications)

## Incretin Therapies

Two naturally occurring hormones (incretins) called GIP and GLP-1 have been identified and are released by cells in the GI tract in response to food. Agents that mimic the actions of incretin hormones may be beneficial therapeutic options.

Exenatide (Byetta), a GLP-1 receptor agonist given *subcutaneously* twice daily, mimics the action of the incretin GLP-1. It also decreases glucagon secretion, delays gastric emptying time, and decreases food intake (increases satiety), resulting in weight loss. Bydureon is a long-acting form of the medication in Byetta and is given subcutaneously once weekly.

Exenatide is indicated as adjunctive therapy for Type 2 patients who have not achieved glycemic control and are taking metformin, a sulfonylurea, or a glitazone.

Common *side effects* include nausea or vomiting, diarrhea, dyspepsia, gastroesophageal reflux, injection site reactions, and hypoglycemia (when given in combination with sulfonylureas). It is not recommended for use in patients with severe renal disease or a history of pancreatitis.

Sitagliptin (Januvia), saxagliptin (Onglyza) and linagliptin (Tradjenta), given *orally* once daily, are indicated for use as monotherapy in Type 2 patients or in combination with other agents when adequate glycemic control has not been achieved and may be preferred agents in older adults.

Common *side effects* include abdominal pain, diarrhea, nausea, vomiting, upper respiratory tract infection, and nasopharyngitis. Use these agents with caution (if at all) in patients with a history of pancreatitis. Dosage adjustments are required for renal disease (except for linagliptin).

## Meglitinides

Nateglinide (Starlix) and repaglinide (Prandin) stimulate the beta cells of the pancreas to produce insulin. They can be used as monotherapy or in combination with metformin. Meglitinides have a rapid onset and short duration of action, and are to be taken before each meal.

Side effects of meglitinides may include:

- GI effects (nausea or vomiting, diarrhea, constipation, dyspepsia, and abdominal cramps)
- Hypoglycemia; initial weight gain
- Upper respiratory infection (URI), sinusitis, arthralgia, and headache

Precautions or contraindications for meglitinides apply to:

Diabetic ketoacidosis

Impaired liver function

Pregnancy and lactation

Children

Drug interactions with meglitinides include (refer to the listing under sulfonylureas):

Administer before meals to maximize absorption

Gemfibrozil (Lopid) may enhance or prolong effects

## Thiazolidinediones

Pioglitazone (Actos) and rosiglitazone (Avandia) lower blood glucose by decreasing insulin resistance and improving sensitivity to insulin in muscle, liver, and adipose tissue. They can be used as monotherapy or concomitantly with other agents.

Product labeling for both pioglitazone and rosiglitazone includes black box warnings regarding the potential for these agents to cause or exacerbate congestive heart failure in some patients, and both are contraindicated with class III or IV heart failure. In addition, a black box warning for the potential increase in the risk of myocardial ischemia has been added to rosiglitazone's label, although the warning also states that the data concerning the increased risk of myocardial ischemia are inconclusive.

Side effects of thiazolidinediones may include:

- Weight gain, fluid retention, and edema (Report weight gain over 6.6 lb, sudden onset of edema, or shortness of breath.)
- URI, sinusitis, pharyngitis, and headache

    Myalgia; atypical bone fractures (upper arm, hand, and foot)
Anemia

    Hypoglycemia (in combination with insulin or oral hypoglycemics)

**Precautions or contraindications** for thiazolidinediones apply to:

Impaired liver function

Heart failure (causes edema); pulmonary edema

May cause resumption of ovulation in premenopausal patients, increasing the risk for pregnancy

Pregnancy and lactation

Children

**Drug interactions** occur between thiazolidinediones and:

Insulins (increase the probability of weight gain, fluid retention, and CHF)

Pioglitazone with oral contraceptives (reduced effectiveness of the contraceptive)

Rosiglitazone with nitrates (increased risk of myocardial ischemia)

"Azole" antifungals (potentiation of hypoglycemic effect)

See Table 23-4 for a summary of the oral hypoglycemics.

**TABLE 23-4** Oral and Injectable Noninsulin Antidiabetic Agents

| GENERIC NAME | TRADE NAME | USUAL DOSAGE |
|---|---|---|
| **First-Generation Sulfonylureas** | | |
| chlorpropamide | | 100–500 mg per day with meal (do not use for older adults) |
| tolbutamide | | 250–3,000 mg per day or divided |
| **Second-Generation Sulfonylureas** | | |
| glimepiride | Amaryl | 1–8 mg per day with meal |
| glipizide | Glucotrol | 2.5–40 mg per day ac or divided |
| | Glucotrol XL | 5–20 mg per day with meal |
| glyburide | Diabeta | 1.25–20 mg per day or divided with meal |
| | Glynase (micronized) | 1.5–12 mg per day with meal |
| **Alpha-Glucosidase Inhibitors** | | |
| acarbose | Precose | 25–100 mg TID, with first bite of meal |
| miglitol | Glyset | |

*(continued)*

**TABLE 23-4** Oral and Injectable Noninsulin Antidiabetic Agents—(*continued*)

| GENERIC NAME | TRADE NAME | USUAL DOSAGE |
|---|---|---|
| **Biguanides** | | |
| metformin | Glucophage | 500–2,550 mg per day divided with meals |
| | Glucophage XR | 500–2,000 mg per day with P.M. meal or divided |
| **Incretin Therapies** | | |
| *GLP-1 receptor agonist* | | |
| exenatide | Byetta | *subcu* 5–10 mcg BID ac (A.M. & P.M. meal) |
| | Bydureon | *subcu* 2 mg weekly (any time of day) |
| *DPP-4 inhibitors ("gliptins")* | | |
| linagliptin | Tradjenta | PO 5 mg daily |
| sitagliptin | Januvia | PO 50–100 mg daily |
| saxagliptin | Onglyza | PO 2.5–5 mg daily |
| **Meglitinides** | | |
| nateglinide | Starlix | 60–120 mg TID ac |
| repaglinide | Prandin | 0.5–4 mg BID two to four times per day ac |
| **Thiazolidinediones** | | |
| pioglitazone | Actos | 15–45 mg per day |
| rosiglitazone | Avandia | 4–8 mg per day or BID divided (restricted access/distribution) |
| **Combinations** | | |
| glyburide/metformin | Glucovance | 1.25/250–20/2,000 mg per day or BID with meals |
| rosiglitazone/metformin | Avandamet | 2/500–8/2,000 mg per day with meals or divided (restricted access/distribution) |
| sitagliptin/metformin | Janumet | 50/500–50/1,000 mg BID with meals |

*Note:* In older adults, start with the lowest dose possible and titrate upward to achieve desired glycemic control.

# PATIENT EDUCATION

Patients with both Type 1 and Type 2 diabetes should be instructed regarding:

Prevention of hypoglycemia—the importance of control with proper drug and diet therapy and *never* skipping meals; do not consume alcohol on an empty stomach.

Early symptoms and treatment of hypoglycemia—carrying a ready source of carbohydrate (e.g., glucose tablets, lump sugar, or candy); orange juice, 4 oz, is also appropriate

Properly balanced diet (i.e., restricted calories); avoidance of simple sugars, alcohol, and foods high on the Glycemic Index (e.g., white bread, white potatoes, and white rice).

Substitute foods low on the Glycemic Index—complex carbohydrates, such as whole-grain breads and cereal and brown rice. Reduce fats, increase fiber, and be sure to have an adequate fluid intake.

Regular exercise and maintenance of proper body weight; weight reduction if obese

Importance of reporting to a physician *immediately* if nausea, vomiting, diarrhea, or infections occur (IV fluids may be required to prevent dehydration and acidosis)

Good foot care to reduce the chance of infections

Carrying identification card and wearing identification tag

Look-alike, sound-alike drugs: Actos/Actonel, glipizide/glyburide, insulin name pairs mentioned earlier

Taking the medication (oral or insulin) at approximately the same time each day and in proper relation to meals

Proper use of monitoring devices; check blood glucose as directed by the physician, especially with hypoglycemia or stress

For patients with Type 1 diabetes (those requiring insulin), the foregoing instructions are important, as well as these additional rules:

Rotate injection sites (Figure 23-2). Insulin is absorbed more rapidly in the arm or thigh, especially with exercise. Inject insulin into abdomen if possible for most consistent absorption.

Maintain aseptic technique with injections.

Have someone check the amount of insulin in the syringe or pen before injection, especially with older adults or those with vision impairment (retinal problems are common in diabetics).

Check all insulin for the expiration date.

Check regular insulin for clearness; do *not* give if cloudy or discolored.

Rotate isophane insulin vials to mix contents; do *not* give if solution is clear or clumped in appearance after rotation; do not shake the vial; rotate gently between hands (Figure 23-3).

If regular insulin is to be mixed with NPH, draw regular insulin into syringe first.

Unopened vials of insulin should be stored at 2–8°C and should not be subjected to freezing. The vial or pen in use may be stored at room temperature for a limited amount of time (depending on the product) without loss of potency.

Avoid exposure of insulin to extremes in temperature or direct sunlight. Do not put vial in glove compartment, trunk, or suitcase.

Regular insulin is sometimes administered as correction for elevated blood glucose readings as ordered by a physician.

Proper disposal of injectable products.

Notify the physician of illness, increased stress, or trauma. *More* insulin may be required under these circumstances.

Notify the physician if you increase your exercise significantly or if you are taking less than the usual amount of food. *Less* insulin may be required under these circumstances.

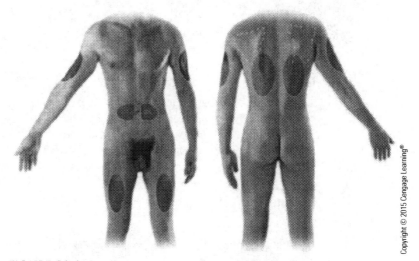

**FIGURE 23-2** Common sites for insulin injection. Sites should be rotated and the site recorded each time on the medication record.

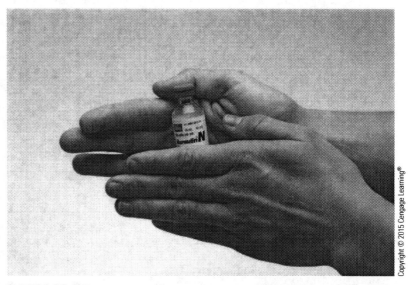

**FIGURE 23-3** Rotate isophane and zinc insulin vials gently to mix contents. Do not shake.

# CASE STUDY A

## ENDOCRINE SYSTEM DRUGS

After weeding in her garden, Marie Kilcline experiences a severe allergic reaction to poison ivy. She presents to her physician with a rash on her face, arms, and legs.

1. The physician prescribes a corticosteroid. How will this category of medication be most beneficial to Marie?
   a. As an antipruritic
   b. As an antineoplastic
   c. As an antidiabetic
   d. As an anti-inflammatory

2. The physician explains that side effects of the corticosteroid may include:
   a. Hypotension
   b. Hypoglycemia
   c. Increased susceptibility to infection
   d. Flushing of the hands and face

3. Prior to handing Marie her prescription, the physician reviews her medication history. He knows this is essential because of possible interactions with corticosteroids. Which drug may cause an interaction resulting in reduced effectiveness of the corticosteroid?
   a. Estrogen
   b. Salicylates
   c. Diuretics
   d. Phenytoin

4. When Marie picks up her corticosteroid medication at the pharmacy, she reads the label on the side of the bottle containing instructions on when to take her medication. Which of the following is most likely to be on this label?
   a. Take 1h before meals.
   b. Avoid taking with milk.
   c. Take 1h after meals.
   d. Take 2h after meals.

5. Marie will be taking her medication for a prescribed amount of time. What will be the best method to discontinue her corticosteroid?
   a. Slowly taper the dosage.
   b. Stop the medication abruptly.
   c. Reduce the dose in alternating weeks.
   d. Administer an IV bolus and then discontinue the medication.

# CASE STUDY B

## ANTIDIABETIC AGENTS

Forty-eight-year-old Marcus Wales has been diagnosed with new onset of Type 2 diabetes. His physician orders a low-fat, low-calorie diet. In addition to dietary changes, the physician would like to start him on an oral hypoglycemic drug.

1. The physician starts him on glyburide, a sulfonylurea medication. He explains to Marcus that sulfonylureas work by:
   a. Blocking glucose uptake into the cell
   b. Increasing insulin production from the pancreas
   c. Decreasing glucagon secretion
   d. Promoting urinary excretion of excess glucose

2. The physician explains to Marcus that one of the side effects of a sulfonylurea medication is:
   a. Insomnia                          c. Excessive urination
   b. Orthostatic hypotension           d. Fatigue

3. Prior to prescribing the medication, the physician reviews Marcus's medical history. This is because sulfonylureas must be used with extreme caution in individuals who:
   a. Are obese                         c. Have impaired kidney and liver function
   b. Are asthmatic                     d. Have peripheral vascular disease

4. The physician cautions Marcus to call him prior to taking any other medication because of possible interactions. Which drug can potentiate the hypoglycemic effect of a sulfonylurea?
   a. Quinolones                        c. Antacids
   b. Penicillins                       d. Rifampin

5. What drug causes an interaction with sulfonylureas, resulting in an antagonistic action in which a larger dose may be required?
   a. MAOIs                             c. Corticosteroids
   b. Testosterone                      d. Narcotic analgesics

# CHAPTER REVIEW QUIZ

Match the medication in the first column with the appropriate classification in the second column. Classifications may be used more than once.

### Medication

1. _____ Glucophage
2. _____ prednisone
3. _____ Humulin R
4. _____ Synthroid
5. _____ Avandia
6. _____ Tapazole
7. _____ Isophane
8. _____ Prandin
9. _____ Lantus
10. _____ Humalog

### Classification

a. Thyroid agent
b. Antithyroid
c. Oral antidiabetic agent
d. Corticosteroid
e. Insulin–rapid acting
f. Insulin–short acting
g. Insulin–intermediate acting
h. Insulin–long acting

**Choose the correct answer.**

11. A patient who is on a thyroid medication should be monitored for which potential side effect?
    a. Hyperglycemia
    b. Hypotension
    c. Muscle twitching
    d. Shortness of breath

12. Thyroid medication should be taken:
    a. At bedtime with a sip of water
    b. On an empty stomach 30–60 min prior to breakfast
    c. 30–60 min after breakfast
    d. With breakfast.

13. Insulin is administered parenterally because:
    a. It is easier to monitor dosage
    b. It is destroyed in the GI tract
    c. Insulin pills are difficult to swallow
    d. Parenteral dosing is tolerated better

14. In order to prevent a medication error, an insulin dose in a syringe:
    a. Should be color-coded for specific doses
    b. Should be drawn up with the nondominant hand for a better visualization of the dose
    c. Should only be verified by a pharmacist
    d. Should be verified by another clinician

15. What best describes the onset and duration of action of regular insulin?

    a. Delayed onset and short duration
    b. Extended onset and long duration
    c. Rapid onset and short duration
    d. Ultra-rapid onset and very short duration

16. The peak of rapid-acting insulins falls under which time frame postinjection?

    a. 1–2 h
    b. 1–5 h
    c. 6–12 h
    d. 12–24 h

17. What is one of the most likely symptoms of hyperglycemia?

    a. Weight gain
    b. Excitability
    c. Excessive thirst
    d. Urinary retention

18. Which of the following may potentiate the hypoglycemic effect of insulin?

    a. NSAIDs
    b. Corticosteroids
    c. Antidepressants
    d. Alcohol

19. Which preparation of insulin is used to correct elevated blood glucose?

    a. Lispro
    b. Regular
    c. Isophane (NPH)
    d. Glargine

20. Illness, increased stress, or trauma may have what effect on a prescribed dose of insulin?

    a. Less insulin may be required.
    b. The dose will need to be divided.
    c. More insulin may be required.
    d. No change in dosage will be required.

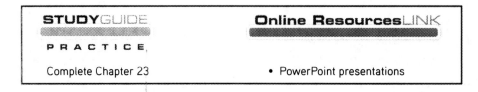

| **STUDY**GUIDE | **Online Resources**LINK |
|---|---|
| **P R A C T I C E** | |
| Complete Chapter 23 | • PowerPoint presentations |

# CHAPTER 25

## CARDIOVASCULAR DRUGS

## Objectives

*Upon completion of this chapter, the learner should be able to*

1. Describe the indication, action, and effects of digoxin and toxic side effects

2. Identify the different types of antiarrhythmics, general indications, side effects, and associated patient education

3. Identify the most commonly used antihypertensives, side effects, and required patient education

4. Describe the different types of coronary vasodilators with cautions, side effects, and patient education

5. Name the six antilipemic categories and describe their actions, common drugs, and patient education

6. Compare and contrast the three categories of antithrombotic agents in terms of administration, action, typical drugs, and antidotes

7. Explain appropriate and important patient education for all categories of antithrombotic therapy

8. Define the Key Terms and Concepts

## Key Terms and Concepts

Antiarrhythmic agents
Anticoagulants
Antihypertensives
Antilipemic agents
Antithrombotic agents
Bradycardia
Cardiac glycosides
Coronary heart disease (CHD)
Coronary vasodilators
Heart failure
Hematopoiesis
Hypertension
Hypotension
Ischemia
Platelet inhibitors
Tachycardia
Thrombolytic agents

Cardiovascular drugs include medications that affect the heart and blood vessels as well as anticoagulant and antiplatelet agents that prevent clotting. The drugs described in this chapter are divided into the following categories: cardiac glycosides, antiarrhythmic agents, antihypertensives, vasodilators, antilipemic agents, anticoagulants, platelet inhibitors, thrombolytics, and hematopoietic agents. Some of the drugs described in this chapter fall into more than one category because of their multiple actions and uses (e.g., propranolol, which is used to treat cardiac arrhythmias, hypertension, and angina). Diuretics, which also affect the blood vessels and reduce blood pressure, are discussed in Chapter 15. Autonomic nervous system effects of these drugs are explained in Chapter 13.

# CARDIAC GLYCOSIDES (DIGOXIN)

Cardiac glycosides occur widely in nature or can be prepared synthetically. These glycosides act directly on the myocardium to increase the force of myocardial contractions. Digoxin is the only clinical drug currently used in the cardiac glycoside family. Cardiac glycosides are used primarily in the treatment of heart failure in patients with symptoms that persist after optimization of treatment with an ACE inhibitor, a beta-adrenergic blocker, and/or a diuretic. They are sometimes also used alone or in conjunction with other medications (such as calcium channel blockers) to *slow* the ventricular response in patients with atrial fibrillation or flutter.

In patients with heart failure, the heart fails to adequately pump nutrients and oxygen to body tissues. Since the heart is failing, the body attempts to compensate by retaining salt and fluid, and this may result in both pulmonary and peripheral edema. The heart increases in size to compensate for the increased work load. Symptoms of heart failure include fatigue, weakness, dyspnea, cyanosis, increased heart rate, cough, and pitting edema. A small percentage of patients with heart failure will go on to develop atrial fibrillation. Two disabling and devastating complications of atrial fibrillation are ischemic stroke and systemic embolism.

In patients with heart failure, the cardiac glycosides act by *increasing the force of the cardiac contractions* without increasing oxygen consumption, thereby increasing cardiac output. Cardiac glycosides also lower norepinephrine levels, which are elevated in heart failure and are toxic to the failing heart. As a result of increased efficiency, the heart beats slower, the heart size shrinks, and the concurrent diuretic therapy decreases edema.

The most commonly used cardiac glycosides are digitalis products. Of these, digoxin (Lanoxin) is the only product still marketed for clinical use because it can be administered orally and parenterally and has an intermediate duration of action.

There is a very narrow margin between effective therapy with digoxin and dangerous toxicity. Careful monitoring of cardiac rate and rhythm with EKG (electrocardiogram), cardiac function, side effects, and serum digoxin levels is required to determine the therapeutic maintenance dose. Checking the apical pulse before administering digoxin is an important part of this monitoring process. If the apical pulse rate is less than 60, digoxin may need to be withheld until the physician is consulted. The action taken should be documented.

Modification of dosage is based on individual requirements and response as determined by general condition, renal function, and cardiac function, monitored by EKG. When changing from tablets or IM therapy to elixir or IV therapy, digoxin dosage adjustments may be required.

Toxic side effects of digoxin, which should be reported to the physician immediately, can include:

- Anorexia, nausea, and vomiting (early signs of toxicity)
  Abdominal cramping, distention, and diarrhea
- Headache, fatigue, lethargy, and muscle weakness
- Vertigo, restlessness, irritability, tremors, and seizures
- Visual disturbances including blurring, diplopia (double vision), or halos

- Cardiac arrhythmias of all kinds, especially bradycardia (rate less than 60)
- Electrolyte imbalance, especially potassium (either hyperkalemia or hypokalemia can cause arrhythmias)
- Insomnia, confusion, and mental disorders, especially with older adults

Treatment of digoxin toxicity includes:

Discontinuing the drug immediately (usually sufficient)

Monitoring electrolytes for hyperkalemia, hypokalemia, hypomagnesemia, and hypercalcemia

Drugs such as atropine for symptomatic bradycardia

Digoxin-specific Fab fragments (DigiFab) as an antidote in life-threatening toxicity

Precautions or contraindications apply to:

Severe pulmonary disease

Hypothyroidism

Acute myocardial infarction, acute myocarditis, and severe heart failure

Impaired renal function; hypokalemia and hypomagnesemia

Arrhythmias not caused by heart failure

Pregnancy and lactation

High doses in older adults

Interactions of digoxin may occur with:

Antacids, cholestyramine, neomycin, and rifampin (reduce the absorption of digoxin; administer far apart)

Diuretics, calcium, and corticosteroids (can increase the chance of arrhythmias)

Macrolides and antiarrhythmics (*especially* quinidine and verapamil; may potentiate digoxin toxicity)

Adrenergics (epinephrine, ephedrine, and isoproterenol; increase the risk of arrhythmias)

## PATIENT EDUCATION

Patients taking digoxin should be instructed regarding:

Recognition and immediate reporting of side effects

Holding medication, if any side effects occur, until the physician can be consulted

Avoiding taking any other medication at the same time without physician approval

Avoiding all over-the-counter (OTC) medication, especially antacids and cold remedies

Avoiding abrupt withdrawal after prolonged use; must be reduced gradually under physician supervision

Checking heart rate (pulse) on a regular basis

# ANTIARRHYTHMIC AGENTS

The term "arrhythmia" refers to any change from the normal sequence of electrical impulses of the heart. The electrical impulses may happen too fast, too slowly, or erratically—causing the heart to beat too fast (tachycardia), too slowly (bradycardia), or erratically (fibrillation). Antiarrhythmic agents include a variety of drugs that act in different ways to suppress various types of cardiac arrhythmias, including atrial or ventricular tachycardias, atrial fibrillation or flutter, and arrhythmias that occur with digoxin toxicity or during surgery and anesthesia. The choice of a particular antiarrhythmic agent is based on the careful assessment of many factors, including the type of arrhythmia; frequency; cardiac, renal, or other pathological condition; and current signs and symptoms.

The role of the health care practitioner is critical in this area in accurate and timely reporting of vital signs, pertinent observations regarding the effectiveness of medications and adverse side effects, and modification of precipitating causes. Adequate knowledge of drug action and effects, along with good judgment, is essential.

Side effects of the individual medications are discussed separately. However, keep in mind that most of the drugs given to counteract arrhythmias have the potential for lowering blood pressure and slowing heartbeat. Therefore, it is especially important to be alert for the signs of hypotension and bradycardia, which could lead to cardiac arrest. Although the antiarrhythmics commonly slow the heart rate, there are exceptions (e.g., procainamide and quinidine, which may cause *tachycardia*). When other cardiac drugs are administered concomitantly, cardiac effects may be additive or antagonistic. Antiarrhythmic agents can worsen existing arrhythmias or cause new arrhythmias, and therefore *careful monitoring is essential.*

Arrhythmia detection or monitoring can include EKG rhythm strips and 24-h Holter monitoring as indicated. Electrolyte surveillance, especially for disorders of potassium and magnesium, is very important for patients on antiarrhythmic agents. Nondrug therapy can include the insertion of a pacemaker or an automatic implantable cardioverter-defibrillator (AICD). The AICD has been widely accepted as the most effective treatment for patients with life-threatening ventricular tachycardia or fibrillation and for patients who have survived a cardiac arrest, and the AICD may also be effective in preventing sudden death in certain patients with heart failure.

## Adenosine

Adenosine (Adenocard) is an injectable antiarrhythmic agent with multiple electrophysiological activities that complicate its placement into a single category. It restores normal sinus rhythm in paroxysmal supraventricular tachycardia (PSVT) by slowing conduction time through the atrioventricular (AV) node. Adenosine also has vasodilatory, antiadrenergic, and negative chronotropic (decrease in rate) properties, which act to decrease cardiac oxygen demand.

Adenosine is equal in effectiveness to diltiazem or verapamil in converting PSVT but is less likely to cause hypotension. Common side effects include facial flushing, lightheadedness, headache, dyspnea, and chest pressure. Adenosine is contraindicated in patients with a second- or third-degree heart block or symptomatic bradycardia (unless a functioning artificial pacemaker is present).

# Amiodarone

Amiodarone (Cordarone) is an oral and injectable antiarrhythmic agent approved for the treatment of refractory life-threatening ventricular arrhythmias. Despite its problematic organ toxicity profile and black box warning, amiodarone is widely used for preventing the recurrence of atrial fibrillation. It is considered a broad-spectrum antiarrhythmic with multiple and complex electrophysiological effects. Amiodarone also relaxes both smooth and cardiac muscle, causing decreases in coronary and peripheral vascular resistance and systolic blood pressure.

Side effects of amiodarone, some of which are severe and potentially fatal, but may be less of a problem with lower doses (i.e., 200–400 mg per day), include:

  Pulmonary fibrosis

  Cardiac arrhythmias, induction or worsening of heart failure, and hypotension

  Nausea or vomiting, constipation, and anorexia

  Hepatitis (rare)

  Hyperthyroidism or hypothyroidism

  Neurotoxicity (tremor, peripheral neuropathy, paresthesias [numbness, tingling, especially in extremities])

  Visual disturbances; optic neuropathy and/or neuritis (may progress to permanent blindness)

  Dermatological reactions, especially photosensitivity (avoid exposure, wear protective clothing)

Precautions or contraindications for amiodarone apply to:

  Patients with a second- or third-degree heart block, marked sinus bradycardia due to severe sinus node dysfunction, and when bradycardia has caused syncope (unless a functioning artificial pacemaker is present); cardiogenic shock

  Patients with thyroid disease (due to the large amount of iodine contained in amiodarone)

  Iodine hypersensitivity

  Older adults (more susceptible to thyrotoxic and neurotoxic adverse effects)

Interactions with amiodarone are numerous and significant, including:

  Certain fluoroquinolones, macrolide antibiotics, systemic azole antifungals (QT prolongation)

  Warfarin (can result in serious or fatal bleeding if warfarin dose is not reduced; effect may persist for months after discontinuation)

Certain antiarrhythmics, digoxin, and phenytoin (amiodarone increases serum concentrations of these drugs)

Protease inhibitors and grapefruit juice (increase amiodarone concentrations); beta-blockers, calcium channel blockers, and lidocaine (additive adverse cardiac effects)

Cholestyramine, phenytoin, and rifampin (serum concentrations of amiodarone are decreased, reducing its pharmacologic effect)

## Beta-Adrenergic Blockers

Beta-adrenergic blockers, for example propranolol (Inderal), are antiarrhythmics, which combat arrhythmias by inhibiting adrenergic (sympathetic) nerve receptors. The action is complex, and the results can include a membrane-stabilizing effect on the heart. Propranolol (Inderal), a nonselective beta-blocker, is effective in the management of some cardiac arrhythmias and less effective with others. It is also used in the treatment of hypertension and some forms of chronic angina. Because it also blocks the $beta_2$ receptors in the lungs, it can lead to bronchospasm. *Low doses* of metoprolol (Lopressor), a selective $beta_1$-antagonist, may be used *with caution* in patients with lung conditions that cause bronchospasm. For additional use of beta-blockers, for example with migraine, see Chapter 13 and Table 13-2.

**LEARNING HINT:** $Beta_1$ receptors are found primarily in the heart and when stimulated cause an increase in the rate and force of contraction. $Beta_2$ receptors are found primarily in the lungs (when stimulated cause relaxation or bronchodilation of airways) and blood vessels (when stimulated cause vasodilation). A useful mnemonic is to think how many hearts you have (one) and how many lungs (two): The class of selective *beta-blockers* therefore would decrease the rate and force of contraction of the heart and if nonselective may also cause bronchospasm and mild vasoconstriction of blood vessels.

Side effects of beta-blockers, especially in patients over 60 years old and more commonly with the IV administration of the drug, can include:

Hypotension, with vertigo and syncope

Bradycardia, with rarely heart block and cardiac arrest

CNS symptoms (usually with long-term treatment with high doses), including dizziness, irritability, confusion, nightmares, insomnia, visual disturbances, weakness, sleepiness, lassitude, or fatigue

GI symptoms, including nausea, vomiting, and diarrhea or constipation

Rash or hematological effects (rare or transient)

⏺ Bronchospasm, especially with a history of asthma

⏺ Hypoglycemia

Impotence (reported rarely)

**Precautions or contraindications** for the beta-blockers apply to:

Withdrawal after prolonged use (should always be gradual)

Withdrawal before surgery (weigh risk vs. benefits)

Diabetes (may cause hypoglycemia and mask the tachycardic response to hypoglycemia)

Renal and hepatic impairment

Asthma and allergic rhinitis (may cause bronchospasm)

Bradycardia, heart block, and congestive heart failure (CHF)

Pediatric use

Pregnancy and lactation

Chronic obstructive pulmonary disease (COPD)

**Interactions** include *antagonism* of beta-blockers by:

Adrenergics (e.g., epinephrine and isoproterenol)

NSAIDs and salicylates

Tricyclic antidepressants

**Potentiation** of the *hypotensive effect* of propranolol occurs with:

Diuretics and other antihypertensives, for example calcium channel blockers

MAOIs; phenothiazine and other tranquilizers

Cimetidine (Tagamet), which slows metabolism of the drug

Certain antiarrhythmic drugs (e.g., adenosine, digoxin, and quinidine), which may potentiate toxic effects

Alcohol, muscle relaxants, and sedatives, which may precipitate hypotension, dizziness, confusion, or sedation

## Calcium Channel Blockers

Of the calcium channel blockers available, only verapamil (Calan) and diltiazem (Cardizem) possess significant antiarrhythmic activity. These agents are indicated for the treatment of atrial fibrillation/flutter and PSVT. Verapamil and diltiazem counteract arrhythmias by slowing AV nodal conduction. Calcium channel blockers are also used in the treatment of angina and hypertension.

**Side effects** of calcium channel blockers can include:

⏺ Hypotension, with vertigo and headache

⏺ Bradycardia, with heart block

⏺ Edema

⏺ Constipation, nausea, and abdominal discomfort

**NOTE**

Do not take grapefruit juice with certain calcium channel blockers since adverse effects may be potentiated.

Precautions or contraindications for calcium channel blockers apply to:

Heart block, heart failure, or angina

Hepatic and renal impairment

Pregnancy and lactation

Children

Hypotension and heart block

Certain arrhythmias and severe heart failure

Interactions of calcium channel blockers with other cardiac drugs, for example digoxin, can potentiate both good and adverse effects.

Antagonistic effects with calcium channel blockers include:

Barbiturates, cimetidine, phenytoin, ranitidine, and rifampin

Hypotensive effect potentiated with diuretics, ACE (angiotensin-converting enzyme) inhibitors, beta-blockers, and quinidine

## Lidocaine

Local anesthetics (e.g., lidocaine) are administered for their antiarrhythmic effects and membrane-stabilizing action. Lidocaine has been historically used as a first-line antiarrhythmic agent for acute, life-threatening ventricular arrhythmias. However, it is now considered a second choice behind other alternative agents (e.g., IV amiodarone) for the treatment of ventricular arrhythmias.

Side effects of lidocaine are usually of short duration, are dose related, and can include:

- CNS symptoms, including tremors, seizures, dizziness, confusion, and blurred vision
- Hypotension, bradycardia, and heart block
- Dyspnea, respiratory depression, and arrest

  EKG monitoring and availability of resuscitative equipment are necessary during the IV administration of lidocaine.

Precautions or contraindications with lidocaine apply to:

Patients hypersensitive to local anesthetics of this type (amide type)

Heart block and respiratory depression

Pregnancy and lactation

Children

Interactions of lidocaine with other cardiac drugs may be additive or antagonistic and may potentiate adverse effects. Other interactions may be of minor clinical significance since lidocaine is usually titrated to response.

# Procainamide

Procainamide, quinidine, and disopyramide (Norpace) are antiarrhythmic agents. They act by decreasing myocardial excitability, inhibiting conduction, and may depress myocardial contractility. These agents possess anticholinergic properties. IV procainamide is a potential treatment alternative (to amiodarone) for the treatment of ventricular tachycardia during CPR. These agents are used orally primarily as prophylactic therapy to maintain normal rhythm after conversion by other methods.

Side effects of this class of antiarrhythmics are numerous and may necessitate cessation of treatment. They may include:

- Diarrhea, anorexia, nausea and vomiting, and abdominal pain (which are common)
- *Tachycardia*, QT prolongation, hypotension, and syncope
- Anticholinergic effects, including dry mouth, blurred vision, confusion, constipation, and urinary retention
- Vascular collapse and respiratory arrest with IV administration
  Vision abnormalities or hearing disturbances (with quinidine)
  Blood dyscrasias, including anemia, clotting deficiencies, and leukopenia (relatively rare)
  Hepatic disorders; fever
- Dermatological effects, including rash, pruritis, urticaria

Precautions or contraindications with these agents apply to:

Atrioventricular block and conduction defects

Electrolyte imbalance

Digoxin toxicity

Heart failure and hypotension

Myasthenia gravis

Older adults—more susceptible to hypotensive and anticholinergic effects

Children

Pregnancy and lactation

Hepatic or renal disorders

Hypersensitivity to "ester-type" local anesthetics with procainamide

Systemic lupus erythematosus (SLE) with procainamide

Interactions with increased possibility of toxicity may occur with:

Muscle relaxants and neuromuscular blockers

Anticholinergics, tricyclic antidepressants, and phenothiazines

Other cardiac drugs, especially digoxin and antihypertensives

Interactions with increased possibility of *quinidine* toxicity may occur with:

Antiretroviral protease inhibitors

Antacids or sodium bicarbonate

Anticonvulsants (e.g., phenytoin and phenobarbital; cause decreased serum levels)

Anticoagulants (action can be potentiated by quinidine)

## Propafenone

Propafenone (Rythmol) is an oral antiarrhythmic agent used to treat symptomatic supraventricular arrhythmias or severe, life-threatening ventricular arrhythmias. It is also useful in converting atrial fibrillation to sinus rhythm and maintaining it. Propafenone has local anesthetic effects, direct stabilizing action on myocardial membranes, and beta-adrenergic blocking properties.

Side effects of propafenone may include:

Dizziness and blurred vision

Nausea, vomiting, unusual taste, and constipation

Angina, heart failure, palpitations, arrhythmia, and dyspnea

Fatigue, weakness, and headache

Rash

Precautions or contraindications include:

Asthma or acute bronchospasm

Second or third-degree heart block (in the absence of a pacemaker), cardiogenic shock, heart failure, and bradycardia

Marked hypotension and electrolyte imbalance

Interactions of propafenone may occur with:

Quinidine, ritonavir, and certain SSRIs (may cause serum levels of propafenone to be elevated)

Beta-blockers, digoxin, and theophylline (may result in increased serum levels of the same)

## PATIENT EDUCATION

Patients taking antiarrhythmics should be instructed regarding:

Immediate reporting of adverse side effects, especially palpitations, irregular or slow heartbeat, faintness, dizziness, weakness, respiratory distress, and visual disturbances

Holding the medication, if there are side effects, until the physician is contacted

Rising slowly from a reclining position

Modification of lifestyle to reduce stress

Mild exercise on a regular basis as approved by the physician

Not discontinuing the medicine, even if the patient feels well

Taking proper dosage of the medication on time, as prescribed, without skipping any dose

If the medication is forgotten, not doubling the dose

Taking the medication with a full glass of water on an empty stomach, 1h before or 2h after meals, so that it will be absorbed more efficiently (unless stomach upset occurs or the physician prescribes otherwise)

Avoiding taking any other medication, including OTC medicines, unless approved by the physician

Discarding expired medicines and renewing the prescription

Avoiding comparisons with other patients on similar drugs

Contacting the physician immediately with any concerns regarding medicines

See Table 25-1 for a summary of cardiac glycosides and the antiarrhythmics.

**TABLE 25-1** Cardiac Glycosides and Antiarrhythmics

| GENERIC NAME | TRADE NAME | DOSAGE | COMMENTS[b] |
|---|---|---|---|
| **Cardiac Glycoside** | | | |
| digoxin | Lanoxin | PO: tablets, elixir, IM, IV, dosage varies | Monitor serum levels (0.5–0.8 mg/mL for heart failure; 0.8 –2 mg/mL for afib) |
| **Antiarrhythmics** | (grouped by class) | | |
| IA procainamide | | IV | For VTach, afib, PAT, PSVT. Has anticholinergic properties |
| IB lidocaine | Xylocaine | IV diluted | Local anesthetic—amide type for Vfib, VTach. Check IV dilution directions |
| IC propafenone | Rythmol | PO, 150–300 mg q8h | For afib, PSVT, VTach |
| | Rythmol SR | PO, 225–425 mg q12h | For afib prevention |
| II metoprolol[a] | Lopressor | PO, 25–100 mg BID | Beta-blocker for heart rate control in afib |
| | | IV, 2.5–5 mg IV bolus, repeat q5 min for three doses total | |
| III amiodarone | Cordarone, Pacerone | IV, PO; dose varies | For ventricular arrhythmias. Also a vasodilator; Medication Guide required |
| IV verapamil[a] | Calan | IV 2.5–10 mg; PO 240–480 mg daily in divided doses | Calcium channel blocker for afib and PSVT |
| adenosine | Adenocard | IV bolus 6 mg; then 12 mg PRN up to 30 mg | For PSVT; do not confuse with amiodarone |

*Note:* Other antiarrhythmics are available. This is a representative sample by classification.

[a]afib = atrial fibrillation; PAT = paroxysmal atrial tachycardia; PSVT = paroxysmal supraventricular tachycardia; Vfib = ventricular fibrillation; VTach = ventricular tachycardia.

[b]Has other cardiac uses.

# ANTIHYPERTENSIVES

Hypertension is a widespread epidemic that affects as many as one billion people worldwide and approximately 65 million adults in the United States. It is defined as systolic blood pressure (SBP) of 140 or greater or diastolic blood pressure (DBP) of 90 or greater. There is a strong, consistent relationship between blood pressure (BP) and the risk of cardiovascular disease (CVD). High blood pressure increases the risk of angina, myocardial infarction, heart failure, stroke, retinopathy, peripheral arterial disease, and kidney disease and thus requires aggressive treatment.

An additional 37% of adults in the United States are considered to have *prehypertension* (SBP range of 120–139 and DBP range of 80–89), a condition that may identify patients who are at a higher cardiovascular risk based on BP and a higher risk for developing sustained hypertension in later years. The purpose of this classification is to encourage patients to initiate or continue healthy lifestyle practices, rather than to begin antihypertensive drug therapy. Such practices include weight reduction (in patients who are overweight and obese), use of the *Dietary Approaches to Stop Hypertension* (DASH) eating plan, dietary sodium reduction, increased physical activity, modified alcohol use, and smoking cessation.

Antihypertensives do not cure hypertension; they only control it. After withdrawal of the drug, BP will return to levels similar to those before treatment with the medication, if all other factors remain the same. If antihypertensive therapy is to be terminated for some reason, the dosage should be gradually reduced, as abrupt withdrawal can cause rebound hypertension.

Drugs given to lower blood pressure act in various ways. The drug of choice varies according to the stage of hypertension (stage one or stage two), other physical factors (especially other cardiac or renal complications), and effectiveness in individual cases. Frequently, antihypertensives are prescribed on a trial basis and then the dosage or medication is changed, and sometimes antihypertensives are combined for greater effectiveness and to reduce side effects. The health care practitioner must be observant of vital signs and side effects in order to assist the physician in the most effective treatment of hypertension on an individual basis.

Side effects of antihypertensives are common. The most common side effect of antihypertensives is *hypotension*, especially postural hypotension. Another side effect common to many of the antihypertensives is *bradycardia*. Exceptions include hydralazine, which can cause tachycardia.

## Thiazide Diuretics

Most patients meeting the criteria for drug therapy should be started on thiazide-type diuretics, either alone or in combination with a drug from one of the other drug classes: ACE inhibitors, angiotensin receptor blockers, beta-blockers, or calcium channel blockers. Thiazide diuretics appear to be as effective as other antihypertensive agents and, in addition, are inexpensive. See Chapter 15 for a detailed discussion of these agents, especially side effects, precautions or contraindications, and interactions.

# Beta-Adrenergic and Calcium Channel Blockers

Like thiazide diuretics, beta-adrenergic blockers such as carvedilol (Coreg) and metoprolol (Lopressor, Toprol XL) are generally well tolerated and are suitable for initial therapy in some patients with angina, postmyocardial infarction, ischemic heart disease, heart failure, and certain arrhythmias. Only bisoprolol, carvedilol, and metoprolol extended-release have been proven to reduce mortality when used in patients with heart failure. Atenolol should not be used to treat hypertension because this drug has no effect in reducing cardiovascular events and mortality.

Calcium channel blockers such as diltiazem (Cardizem) and nifedipine (Procardia) are an initial therapy option for hypertensive patients with diabetes or high coronary disease risk. They are more effective in treating African-American patients, older adults, and patients with higher pretreatment blood pressure readings. They may also be preferred in patients with obstructive airways disease. Based on historical data, *short-acting* calcium channel blockers should never be used to manage *hypertensive crisis* because of the reports of increased risks of myocardial infarction and mortality.

Because of their pharmacology, verapamil and diltiazem may be used to treat various arrhythmias. Refer to the discussion under "Antiarrhythmic Agents" earlier in this chapter for more information on these agents.

# Angiotensin-Converting Enzyme (ACE) Inhibitors (ACEIs)

Another class of antihypertensives is the angiotensin-converting enzyme (ACE) inhibitors, for example lisinopril or enalapril. Inhibition of ACE lowers blood pressure by *decreasing vasoconstriction*; there are not significant changes in heart rate or cardiac output. ACEIs are first- or second-line agents in the treatment of hypertension and are excellent alone, but also effective and synergistic in combination with other antihypertensives, including diuretics and calcium channel blockers.

ACEIs are especially good choices for patients who also have other serious conditions, including those with heart failure, following myocardial infarction, when high coronary disease risk exists, diabetes, renal disease, and cerebrovascular disease. For example, ACEIs can be considered drugs of choice for hypertensive patients with nephropathy because they slow the progression of the renal disease. They are more effective in younger and white populations and less effective in black patients, unless given in higher doses or in combination with a diuretic.

Side effects of ACE inhibitors (infrequent and usually mild) can include:

- Rash or photosensitivity
- Loss of taste perception; metallic taste
- Blood dyscrasias
- Renal impairment
- Severe hypotension
- Chronic dry cough or nasal congestion
- Hyperkalemia (monitor serum potassium levels periodically)

Precautions or contraindications with ACE inhibitors apply to:

   Collagen disease, for example lupus or scleroderma

   Heart failure

   Angioedema

   Pregnancy and lactation

   Children

Interactions of ACE inhibitors apply to:

   Diuretics (potentiate hypotension; watch BP closely)

   Vasodilators (watch BP closely)

   Potassium-sparing diuretics and potassium supplements (hyperkalemia risk)

   Nonsteroidal anti-inflammatory drugs (NSAIDs) and salicylates (antagonize effects of ACE inhibitors and increase deterioration of renal function in patients with compromised renal function)

   Antacids (decrease absorption)

   Digoxin (possible digitalis toxicity)

   Lithium (risk of lithium toxicity)

## Angiotensin Receptor Blockers (ARBs)

Angiotensin receptor blockers (ARBs) are similar to ACE inhibitors (ACEIs) and are generally used as alternatives. They block the angiotensin receptor that causes vasoconstriction when stimulated by angiotensin II. ARBs such as losartan (Cozaar) and valsartan (Diovan) block the effects of angiotensin II, decreasing blood pressure without a marked change in heart rate.

Compared to ACEIs, ARBs are associated with a lower incidence of drug-induced cough, rash, and/or taste disturbances and are used in those patients who cannot tolerate ACEIs. Like the ACEIs, African-American patients experience a smaller antihypertensive response with the ARBs compared to other ethnic populations. The addition of a low-dose thiazide diuretic to an ARB significantly improves hypertensive efficacy. ARBs are also good choices for patients with other serious conditions, including those with heart failure, diabetes, and renal disease.

Side effects are relatively uncommon with ARBs and include dizziness, orthostatic hypotension, upper respiratory tract infections, and hyperkalemia.

Precautions or contraindications for ARBs apply to:

   Renal impairment

   Pregnancy and lactation

   Children

Interactions with ARBs are similar to those seen with ACEIs.

# OTHER ANTIHYPERTENSIVES

## Antiadrenergic Agents

*Clonidine (Catapres)* is a *central-acting* alpha-adrenergic agent, used mainly in the treatment of hypertension. It is available as an oral preparation, a transdermal system, and an injection for epidural use. Clonidine has also been used successfully in a variety of other conditions including ADHD, nicotine/opiate withdrawal, vascular headaches, glaucoma, ulcerative colitis, Tourette's syndrome, and treatment of severe pain in cancer patients.

*Prazosin (Minipress)* is a *peripheral-acting* alpha-adrenergic blocker used primarily to treat hypertension. Other agents in this class are used to treat benign prostatic hyperplasia (BPH). Treatment with alpha-adrenergic blockers once was considered potentially favorable for the management of hypertension in patients with BPH to target both blood pressure and BPH symptoms. However, a study determined that patients treated with the alpha-blocker doxazosin, when compared with those treated with the diuretic chlorthalidone, had an increased risk for stroke and heart failure. Therefore, hypertension should not be managed with an alpha-blocker alone, and BPH symptoms should be managed separately (see Chapter 15 for a discussion on the use of alpha-blockers in BPH).

## Peripheral Vasodilator

*Hydralazine*, a peripheral vasodilator, is sometimes used in the treatment of moderate to severe hypertension, especially in patients with CHF, because it increases the heart rate and cardiac output. The drug is generally used in conjunction with a diuretic and another hypotensive agent, for example a beta-blocker. A fixed-dose combination of isosorbide dinitrate and hydralazine (BiDil) is available for the treatment of heart failure.

Side effects of hydralazine can include:

- *Tachycardia* and palpitations
- Headache and flushing
- Orthostatic hypotension
- GI effects, including nausea, vomiting, diarrhea, and constipation
- Blood abnormalities
- Edema and weight gain

Precautions or contraindications for hydralazine apply to:

- Systemic lupus erythematosus (SLE)
- Renal disease
- Coronary artery disease and rheumatic heart disease
- Pregnancy, usually (however, many regard hydralazine as the antihypertensive of choice during preeclampsia)

See Figure 25-1, which illustrates the various mechanisms to reduce blood pressure and see Table 25-2 for a summary of the classifications and specific drug examples of antihypertensives.

## Drugs Used to Treat Hypertension

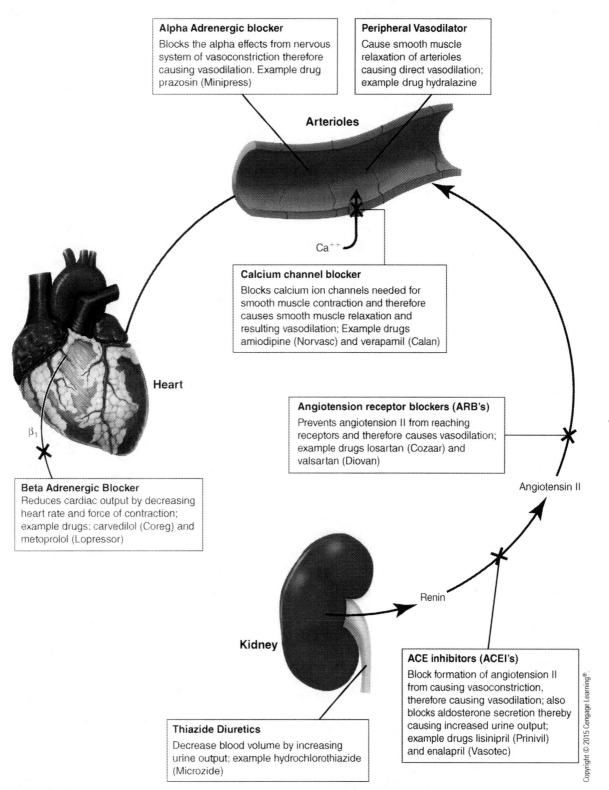

**Alpha Adrenergic blocker**
Blocks the alpha effects from nervous system of vasoconstriction therefore causing vasodilation. Example drug prazosin (Minipress)

**Peripheral Vasodilator**
Cause smooth muscle relaxation of arterioles causing direct vasodilation; example drug hydralazine

**Arterioles**

Ca⁺⁺

**Calcium channel blocker**
Blocks calcium ion channels needed for smooth muscle contraction and therefore causes smooth muscle relaxation and resulting vasodilation; Example drugs amiodipine (Norvasc) and verapamil (Calan)

**Heart**

**Angiotension receptor blockers (ARB's)**
Prevents angiotension II from reaching receptors and therefore causes vasodilation; example drugs losartan (Cozaar) and valsartan (Diovan)

Angiotensin II

β₁

**Beta Adrenergic Blocker**
Reduces cardiac output by decreasing heart rate and force of contraction; example drugs: carvedilol (Coreg) and metoprolol (Lopressor)

Renin

**Kidney**

**ACE inhibitors (ACEI's)**
Block formation of angiotension II from causing vasoconstriction, therefore causing vasodilation; also blocks aldosterone secretion thereby causing increased urine output; example drugs lisinipril (Prinivil) and enalapril (Vasotec)

**Thiazide Diuretics**
Decrease blood volume by increasing urine output; example hydrochlorothiazide (Microzide)

**FIGURE 25-1** Various mechanisms of action of drugs used to treat hypertension.

**TABLE 25-2** Antihypertensives

| GENERIC NAME | TRADE NAME | DOSAGE |
|---|---|---|
| **Beta-Adrenergic Blockers** | | |
| atenolol | Tenormin | 25–100 mg PO daily |
| carvedilol | Coreg | 6.25–25 mg PO BID with food (also has vasodilatory properties) |
| | Coreg CR | 20–80 mg daily with food (SR)[a] |
| metoprolol | Lopressor | 100–400 mg PO daily in divided doses |
| | Toprol XL | 50–100 mg PO daily (SR) |
| nebivolol | Bystolic | 5–40 mg PO daily (also has vasodilatory properties) |
| propranolol | Inderal | 160–480 mg PO daily in two to three divided doses |
| | Inderal LA[a] | 80–160 mg PO daily (SR) |
| **Calcium Channel Blockers** | | |
| amlodipine | Norvasc | 2.5–10 mg PO daily |
| diltiazem | (cap) Cardizem CD (tab) Cardizem LA | 120–360 mg PO daily (SR); regular-release tabs are not approved to treat hypertension |
| | Diltiazem SR | 120–180 mg PO BID (SR) |
| nifedipine | Procardia XL Adalat CC | 30–90 mg PO daily (SR) |
| verapamil | Calan SR, Isoptin SR | 120–240 mg PO one to two times per day (SR) |
| **ACE Inhibitors** | | |
| benazepril | Lotensin | 10–20 mg one to two times per day |
| enalapril | Vasotec | 5–20 mg PO BID |
| lisinopril | Prinivil, Zestril | 5–40 mg PO daily |
| ramipril | Altace | 2.5–20 mg PO one to two divided doses |
| trandolapril | Mavik | 1–4 mg PO daily |
| **Angiotensin Receptor Blockers** | | |
| losartan | Cozaar | 25–100 mg PO one to two divided doses |
| olmesartan | Benicar | 20–40 mg PO daily |
| telmisartan | Micardis | 20–80 mg PO daily |
| valsartan | Diovan | 80–320 mg PO daily |
| **Other Antihypertensives** | | |
| *Antiadrenergic Agents* | | |
| clonidine | Catapres | 0.1–1.2 mg PO daily in divided doses |
| | Catapres TTS | Weekly patch (delivers 0.1–0.3 mg/24 h) |
| prazosin | Minipres | 1–20 mg PO daily in two to three divided doses |
| *Peripheral Vasodilator* | | |
| hydralazine | | 10–50 mg PO two to four times per day; IM, IV dose varies |

*Note:* This is only a representative list of the most commonly used drugs in this category. There are many others and many in combination with a diuretic.

[a]All extended release products (ER/SR) must be swallowed intact! Quick release of the medication can cause the blood pressure to drop suddenly, sending the patient into shock. Caution is advised due to potential confusion with various name extensions designating extended-release formulations (CC, CD, CR, LA, SR, XL).

## PATIENT EDUCATION

Patients taking antihypertensives should be instructed regarding:

Routinely monitoring blood pressure at home, keeping a log of their blood pressure readings, and sharing this information with their physician

Immediate reporting of any adverse side effects, especially slow or irregular heartbeat, dizziness, weakness, breathing difficulty, gastric distress, and numbness or swelling of extremities

Taking the medication on time as prescribed by the physician; *not* skipping a dose or doubling a dose; *not* discontinuing the medicine, even if the patient is feeling well, without consulting the physician first

Rising slowly from a reclining position to reduce lightheaded feeling

Taking care in driving a car or operating machinery if the medication causes drowsiness (ask the physician, nurse, or pharmacist about the specific medication, since medicines differ and individual reactions differ; older people are more susceptible to this effect)

Potentiation of adverse side effects by alcohol, especially dizziness, weakness, sleepiness, and confusion

Reduction or cessation of smoking to help lower blood pressure

Importance of lifestyle modifications, such as exercise, quitting smoking, limiting alcohol usage, and eating a healthy diet in control of blood pressure; following the physician's instructions regarding appropriate diet for the individual, which may include a low-salt or low-sodium or weight-reduction diet if indicated

Avoiding hot tubs and hot showers, which may cause weakness or fainting

Mild exercise on a regular basis as approved by the physician

Always swallowing the extended-release products intact. Quick release of the medication into the system can cause the blood pressure to drop suddenly, causing loss of consciousness and possible shock.

Avoiding grapefruit juice while taking calcium channel blockers, which can increase the risk of hypotension and other adverse cardiac effects.

## CORONARY VASODILATORS

Coronary vasodilators are used in the treatment of angina. When there is insufficient blood supply (ischemia) to a part of the heart, the result is acute pain. The most common form of angina is angina pectoris, chest pain resulting from decreased blood supply to the heart muscle. Obstruction or constriction of the coronary arteries, which supply the heart muscle with oxygenated blood, results in angina pectoris. Vasodilators are administered to dilate these blood vessels (thus increasing myocardial oxygen supply) and stop attacks of angina or reduce the frequency of angina when administered prophylactically. Coronary vasodilators used in the treatment and prophylactic management of angina include nitrates, beta-blockers, and calcium channel blockers.

The nitrates used most commonly for relief of acute angina pectoris, as well as for long-term prophylactic management, are nitroglycerin and isosorbide (e.g., Isordil, Imdur). Nitroglycerin is available in several forms and can be administered in sublingual tablets allowed to dissolve under the tongue or a sublingual spray for the relief of acute angina pectoris. If chest pain is not relieved or worsens 5 min after a dose, EMS should be activated because unrelieved chest pain can indicate an acute myocardial infarction.

Although the traditional recommendation is for patients to take up to three SL nitroglycerin doses over 15 min *before* accessing the emergency system, recent guidelines suggest an alternative strategy to reduce delays in emergency care. New guidelines recommend instructing a patient with a prior prescription for nitroglycerin to call 911 immediately if chest discomfort or pain is persistent or worsened 5 min after *one* dose of nitroglycerin. Self-treatment with nitrates has been identified as a factor resulting in delays in emergency evaluation.

Nitroglycerin is also available in timed-release capsules and tablets and in an injectable formulation that must be diluted carefully according to the manufacturer's instructions for IV administration. Nitroglycerin tablets and capsules must be stored *only in glass containers* with tight-fitting metal screw tops away from heat. Plastic containers can absorb the medication, and air, heat, or moisture can cause loss of potency. Impaired potency of the SL tablets can be detected by the patient if there is an absence of the tingling sensation under the tongue common to this form of administration.

For the long-term prophylactic management of angina pectoris, nitroglycerin is frequently applied topically as a transdermal system. One type of nitroglycerin that is absorbed through the skin is Nitro-Bid ointment, applied with an applicator-measuring (Appli-Ruler) paper. Usual dosage is 0.5–2 inches applied every 8 h. *Remove old paper first.* The ointment is spread lightly (not massaged or rubbed) over any hairless skin area, and the applicator paper is taped in place. Care must be taken to avoid touching the ointment when applying (accidental absorption through the skin of the fingers can cause headache). If nitroglycerin ointment is discontinued, the dose and frequency must be decreased gradually to prevent sudden withdrawal reactions. See Figure 9-1 in Chapter 9, "Administration," for ointment application technique.

Another topical nitroglycerin product, which has a longer action, is in transdermal form (e.g., Nitro-Dur). The skin patch is applied every 24h (on in A.M./off 12h later in the P.M.) to clean, dry, hairless areas of the upper arm or body. Do not apply below the elbow or knee. *The sites should be rotated* to avoid skin irritation, and raw, scarred, or callused areas should be avoided. Patch dosage varies widely, from 0.1 to 0.8 mg/h daily. *Check prescribed dosage carefully. Remove old patch.*

Another nitrate used for the acute relief of angina pectoris and for the prophylactic long-term management is isosorbide. It is available in SL tablets, regular-release tablets, and timed-release capsules and tablets. When using long-acting nitrates, a 12–14h nitrate-free interval between the last dose of the day and the first dose of the following day is recommended to lessen the risk of nitrate tolerance.

Side effects of the nitrates can include:

- Headache (usually diminishes over time; analgesics may be given to alleviate pain)
- Postural hypotension, including dizziness, weakness, and syncope (*patients should be sitting during the administration of fast-acting nitrates*)

Transient flushing

Rash and skin irritation with transdermal forms

- Blurred vision and dry mouth (discontinue the drug with these symptoms)
- Hypersensitivity reactions, enhanced by alcohol, including nausea, vomiting, diarrhea, cold sweats, tachycardia, and syncope

Precautions or contraindications for nitrates apply to:

Glaucoma

GI hypermotility or malabsorption (with timed-release forms)

Intracranial pressure

Severe anemia

Hypotension

Interactions of nitrates may occur with alcohol, which potentiates hypotensive effects. Phosphodiesterase (PDE) inhibitors such as sildenafil (Viagra), used for erectile dysfunction, are contraindicated in men taking nitrates. The two drugs interact to cause a large, sudden, dangerous drop in blood pressure.

For the long-term prophylactic treatment of angina pectoris, beta-blockers such as metoprolol (Lopressor) and calcium channel blockers such as diltiazem (Cardizem) and verapamil (Calan) are frequently used (see "Antiarrhythmic Agents" for information on side effects, etc.). See Figure 25-2, which illustrates drugs used to treat angina.

# PATIENT EDUCATION

Patients receiving coronary vasodilators (nitrates) should be instructed regarding:

Administering fast-acting preparations (sublingual tablets or spray) while sitting down because the patient may become lightheaded

Rising slowly from a reclining position

Not drinking alcohol or taking PDE inhibitors while taking these medicines, which can cause a serious drop in blood pressure

Using timed-release capsules or tablets to prevent attacks (they work too slowly to help once an attack has started)

The fact that nitrates taken for chronic angina may require periods of drug-free intervals to avoid the development of nitrate tolerance and lessening of antianginal effects

Taking timed-release capsules or tablets on an empty stomach with a full glass of water

Allowing sublingual tablets to dissolve under the tongue or in the cheek pouch and not chewing or swallowing them

Repeating sublingual tablets or spray in 5–10 min for a maximum of three tablets or sprays (if no relief or worsening of chest pain within 5 min after the first tablet, activate EMS, or if EMS is unavailable, report to the emergency department); for patients known to have frequent angina, physicians may provide individualized instructions for the use of SL nitroglycerin, based on the characteristics of the patient's angina, time course, and response to the treatment

Not discontinuing the medication suddenly if administered for several weeks (dosage must be reduced gradually under the physician's supervision)

Sensations to be expected, including facial flushing, headache for a short time, and lightheadedness upon rising too suddenly (if these symptoms persist or become more severe, or other symptoms occur, such as irregular heartbeat or blurred vision, notify the physician at once)

Preventing attacks of angina by administering a sublingual tablet or spray before physical exertion or emotional stress (it is preferable to avoid physical or emotional stress when possible)

See Chapter 9 for patient education regarding the administration of nitroglycerin ointment or patch.

## Drugs Used to Treat Angina

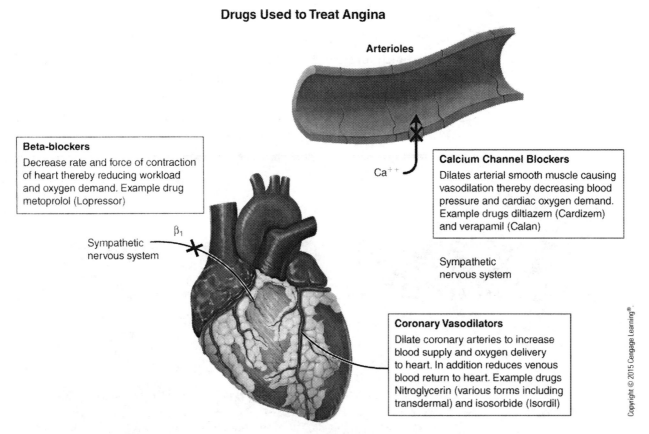

**Arterioles**

**Beta-blockers**
Decrease rate and force of contraction of heart thereby reducing workload and oxygen demand. Example drug metoprolol (Lopressor)

**Calcium Channel Blockers**
Dilates arterial smooth muscle causing vasodilation thereby decreasing blood pressure and cardiac oxygen demand. Example drugs diltiazem (Cardizem) and verapamil (Calan)

$Ca^{++}$

Sympathetic nervous system

$\beta_1$

Sympathetic nervous system

**Coronary Vasodilators**
Dilate coronary arteries to increase blood supply and oxygen delivery to heart. In addition reduces venous blood return to heart. Example drugs Nitroglycerin (various forms including transdermal) and isosorbide (Isordil)

**FIGURE 25-2** Various mechanisms of action of drugs used to treat angina.

See Table 25-3 for a summary of coronary vasodilators.

**TABLE 25-3** Coronary Vasodilators

| GENERIC NAME | TRADE NAME | DOSAGE |
|---|---|---|
| **Nitrates**[a] | | |
| nitroglycerin | Nitrostat tabs S.L. | 1–3 tabs q5min × 3 max in 15 min PRN |
| | Nitrolingual spray | 1–2 sprays (0.4–0.8 mg) SL q5min × 3 max in 15 min PRN |
| | caps E.R. | 2.5–9 mg PO q8–12h |
| | Nitro-Bid oint 2% | 1–2 inches q6–8h (while awake and at bedtime for a 10–12h nitrate-free interval); Note: 1 g unit dose foilpac equiv to ~1" |
| | Nitro-Dur, Minitran | 1 transdermal patch to deliver 0.1–0.8 mg/h daily, rotate site; on 12–14h per off 10–12h |
| | IV, premixed or sol for inj | IV dose varies |
| isosorbide dinitrate | | SL 2.5–5 mg × 3 max in 15–30 min |
| | Isordil | Prophylactic PO 10–40 mg BID–TID (allow for a 14 h nitrate-free interval) |
| | Dilatrate (SR) | PO 40 mg one to two times per day (18 h nitrate-free interval recommended) |
| with hydralazine | BiDil | PO 1–2 tabs TID (for heart failure) |
| isosorbide mononitrate | Imdur (SR) | 10–20 mg PO BID (7 h apart) or TID at 8 A.M., 1 P.M., and 6 P.M. |
| | | 30–120 mg PO one time per day |

*Note:* Beta-blockers and calcium channel blockers are also administered prophylactically for angina pectoris and can be given concurrently with the nitrates.
[a]For the prevention and treatment of angina pectoris.

# ANTILIPEMIC AGENTS

It is estimated that nearly 50% of Americans have elevated total blood cholesterol levels above 200 mg/dL—a key risk factor for coronary heart disease (CHD). Cardiovascular disease is the leading killer of men and women in the United States (more deaths than cancer, diabetes, accidents, and chronic lung diseases combined). High cholesterol can lead to arterial blockage, hardening of the arteries, blood clots, heart attack, or stroke and may even play a role in dementia.

Lipoproteins are responsible for transporting cholesterol and other fats through the blood stream. *Low-density lipoproteins* (LDLs; "bad cholesterol") carry the largest amount of the cholesterol in the blood and are responsible for transporting and depositing it in the arterial walls. *Very low-density lipoproteins* (VLDLs; triglycerides) are precursors of the LDL and compose the largest proportion of lipids in the diet, adipose tissue, and the blood. Triglycerides (TGs) are a source of energy; excess dietary calories are converted to TGs and stored as fat in the adipose tissue for future energy needs. Excess TGs (greater than the normal 150 level) can be an independent risk factor leading to atherosclerosis and CHD, as well as pancreatitis.

*High-density lipoproteins* (*HDLs;* "good cholesterol") help transport LDL cholesterol from the walls of the arteries through the bloodstream to the liver for excretion. An HDL level of below 40 mg/dL is considered low, and each 1 mg/dL increase in the HDL level is associated with a 6% lower risk of cardiovascular disease. LDL cholesterol is the primary target of treatment in clinical lipid management. The use of therapeutic lifestyle changes (TLCs), including LDL-lowering dietary management (e.g., restriction of saturated and trans fats or cholesterol intake, including fiber and soy protein in diet), weight control, appropriate exercise, limiting alcohol intake, and smoking cessation, will achieve the therapeutic goal (LDL below 100 mg/dL) in many persons. If these measures are inadequate, drug therapy may be added. Drug therapy aimed at reducing cholesterol levels either reduces hepatic production or intestinal absorption of cholesterol. Six categories of antilipemic agents used to lower blood cholesterol levels are available: HMG-CoA reductase inhibitors (the *statins*), bile acid sequestrants, nicotinic acid (niacin), fibric acid derivatives, cholesterol absorption inhibitor, and omega-3 fatty acids.

## Statins

HMG-CoA reductase inhibitors (statins) inhibit the enzyme for cholesterol synthesis. These agents are the most potent lipid-lowering medications available for monotherapy and are considered to be the first choice in managing high cholesterol. Statins (e.g., atorvastatin—Lipitor; simvastatin—Zocor) have been shown to be very effective in lowering LDL levels (up to 60%) and are modestly effective in reducing TG levels and increasing HDL levels, thereby reducing cardiovascular morbidity and mortality. Statins are generally well tolerated.

Since HMG-CoA is most active at night when dietary intake is low, most statins are generally given at bedtime in order to provide optimal decreases in LDL levels. Due to their longer half-lives, atorvastatin and rosuvastatin can be given at the same time each day, any time of day. Recently, the maximum dose of simvastatin was reduced from 80 to 40 mg (if using it for less than 12 months) because of the increased risk of myopathy from the higher dose.

Side effects of statins include:

Mild GI disturbances, headache, rash, fatigue

Myalgia and muscle weakness (can try switching to a different statin if problematic)

Rhabdomyolysis (destruction of the muscle tissue leading to renal failure; reported rarely)

Elevated liver enzymes (the FDA recently revised statin labeling by removing the recommendation for periodic liver function tests; baseline tests are still suggested, but follow-up monitoring is necessary only if clinically indicated)

Increased risk (9% to 13%) of new-onset diabetes mellitus with high-dose statin use (benefits of statin therapy far outweigh the risk of statin-induced diabetes; be considerate of the risk and monitor the patient)

Precautions or contraindications for statins apply to:

Hepatic or renal disease

Existing myalgia or muscle weakness

Pregnancy and breast-feeding

Children

Gemfibrozil, HIV, and hepatitis C protease inhibitors (increased risk for myopathy and rhabdomyolysis)

Interactions of certain statins with amiodarone, dronedarone, immunosuppressive drugs, erythromycin, azole antifungals, diltiazem, verapamil, *grapefruit juice*, or other antilipemic drugs (fibrates and niacin) increase the risk of myopathy and renal failure. Recently, the maximum recommended dose for most statins, when taken with certain interacting drugs, was also reduced due to safety considerations.

## Bile Acid Sequestrants

Cholestyramine (Questran) and colesevelam (WelChol), which are not absorbed from the GI tract, bind bile acids in the intestine, interrupting the process by which bile acids are returned to the liver for reuse. Since bile acids are formed from cholesterol, sequestrants reduce total body cholesterol. Bile acid sequestrants can be used as monotherapy when moderate reductions in LDL levels are required or as an add-on therapy to statins. They should not be used as a single agent in the presence of elevated TGs.

Side effects of bile acid sequestrants include:

Constipation, gas, cramps, heartburn, nausea, anorexia, abdominal pain, and bloating (occurs frequently and may affect compliance)

Colesevelam is administered at lower doses because of its higher bile-binding capacity and is associated with fewer GI adverse effects.

Precautions or contraindications for bile acid sequestrants apply to:

Biliary cirrhosis and obstruction

GI obstruction or fecal impaction

Interactions with bile acid sequestrants can reduce the absorption of many drugs, including antibiotics, cardiac glycosides, fat-soluble vitamins, thiazide diuretics, and thyroid hormones (administer at least 1h before or 4h after the bile acid sequestrants).

## Nicotinic Acid (Niacin)

Nicotinic acid reduces the hepatic synthesis of TGs and inhibits the mobilization of free fatty acids from the peripheral tissues. It lowers total and LDL cholesterol and TG levels in the serum and also raises HDL cholesterol levels. Niacin may be useful in combination with a statin in patients with diabetic dyslipidemia (abnormal levels of various blood lipid fractions).

Side effects of niacin can be troublesome and include:

- GI upset, dyspepsia (indigestion), blurred vision, and fatigue
- *Skin flushing*, itching, and irritation (more common with immediate-release preparations; pretreatment with aspirin or ibuprofen can diminish cutaneous reactions)
- Glucose intolerance and hyperuricemia (abnormal uric acid levels in blood) (higher doses)
- Hepatotoxicity (especially with sustained-release products; monitoring hepatic function is recommended for all niacin formulations)

Precautions or contraindications of niacin include:

Hepatic, gallbladder, or peptic ulcer disease; diabetes; glaucoma; or gout

Pregnancy and lactation (high doses)

Children (<10 years old)

Interactions of niacin occur with:

Antihypertensives and vasodilators (potentiate hypotensive effects)

Antidiabetic agents with the loss of blood glucose control

Alcohol (worsens flushing)

> **NOTE**
>
> Regular- and extended-release formulations of niacin are not bioequivalent and are not interchangeable.

## Fibric Acid Derivatives (Fibrates)

The fibrates fenofibrate (TriCor) and gemfibrozil (Lopid) possess minimal LDL-reducing capacity but are especially effective in patients who have extremely high TG levels and elevated cholesterol levels, and in patients with combined forms of hyperlipidemia. They are a good choice for diabetics because they improve glucose tolerance. The mechanism by which fibrates reduce TGs is poorly understood. Fibrates may be used in combination with other antilipemics, since these agents appear to be additive in lowering LDL and raising HDL cholesterol. Fibrates are generally well tolerated.

Side effects of fibrates can include:

- GI complaints (diarrhea, dyspepsia, nausea and vomiting, and abdominal pain)
- Cholethiasis (gallstones in the gallbladder) due to the increased biliary excretion of cholesterol, jaundice, blood dyscrasias, myopathy (abnormal condition of skeletal muscles)
- Hypersensitivity reactions (rare)
- Increased risk of pulmonary emboli (PE)

Precautions or contraindications for fibrates apply to:

Gallbladder, hepatic, renal disease, or peptic ulcer

Pregnancy and lactation

Children

Gemfibrozil with statins (increased risk for myopathy and rhabdomyolysis)

Interactions of fibrates occur with:

Oral anticoagulants and hypoglycemic agents (potentiate effects)

Statins to increase the risk of serious muscle problems and elevated liver enzymes (use together only in the lowest effective doses and if benefits outweigh risks)

Ezetimibe is not advised (increased risk of cholethiasis)

## Cholesterol Absorption Inhibitor

Ezetimibe (Zetia) moderately reduces LDL levels by inhibiting intestinal absorption of both dietary and biliary cholesterol, blocking its transport in the small intestine. It can be taken simultaneously with a statin (Vytorin, a combination product), allowing for lower doses of the statin to be used, and the LDL-lowering effects of the two drugs are additive. Ezetimibe is generally well tolerated, with abdominal pain, back pain, and arthralgia being reported. Patients with gallbladder disease and moderate to severe hepatic insufficiency should not take it.

Administer ezetimibe at least 1 to 2h before or 2 to 4h after administering antacids and bile acid sequestrants, respectively. Avoid use with cyclosporine (increases serum concentrations of both drugs) and fibrates (increased risk of cholethiasis).

## Omega-3 Fatty Acids

Omega-3 fatty acids include eicosapentaenoic acid (EPA) and docosahexaenoic acid (DHA), found in fatty cold-water fish, and alpha-linolenic acid (ALA), found in flaxseed, tofu, soybean oil, canola oil, and nuts. There is evidence that EPA and DHA may have a role in the prevention of primary and secondary heart disease and reduce TGs (as an adjunct to diet or simvastatin).

The best source of omega-3 fatty acids is fatty fish, like salmon, but fish oil capsules may be more convenient, especially if high doses are needed. A highly concentrated and purified form of omega-3 fatty acids is also available by prescription only as *Lovaza*. Fish oil can cause nausea, heartburn, or diarrhea. A fishy aftertaste can be reduced by refrigeration or freezing (Lovaza should not be frozen). Since omega-3 fatty acids inhibit platelet aggregation, caution is advised when used concurrently with anticoagulants, platelet inhibitors, and thrombolytic agents. The DHA component of omega-3 fatty acids may be responsible for the elevations in LDL levels seen with these products; patients should be monitored to ensure their LDL levels do not increase excessively.

See Table 25-4 for a summary of antilipemic agents.

**TABLE 25-4** Antilipemic Agents

| GENERIC NAME | TRADE NAME | DOSAGE |
|---|---|---|
| **Antilipemic Agents** | | |
| *Statins* | | |
| atorvastatin | Lipitor | 10–80 mg PO daily |
| lovastatin | Mevacor | 20–80 mg PO at bedtime with food |
| pravastatin | Pravachol | 10–80 mg PO at bedtime |
| rosuvastatin | Crestor | 5–40 mg PO daily |
| simvastatin | Zocor | 5–40 mg PO at bedtime (80 mg if already on it with no evidence of myopathy) |
| *Bile Acid Sequestrants* | | |
| cholestyramine | Questran, Questran Light | 4 g one to two times per day ac; mix powder with water, milk, or juice |
| colesevelam | Welchol | 6 tabs (625 mg each) daily or 3 tabs BID with food and a full glass of water; max 7 tabs per day |
| *Nicotinic Acid* | | |
| niacin | Niaspan (Rx) Slo-Niacin (OTC) | Dose varies with response; take after meals or a snack |
| *Fibric Acid Derivatives* | | |
| fenofibrate | Antara, Lofibra, Tricor, Trilipix | 43–200 mg PO daily with food depending on formulation/ manufacturer |
| gemfibrozil | Lopid | 600 mg PO BID ac |
| *Cholesterol Absorption Inhibitor* | | |
| ezetimibe | Zetia | 10 mg PO daily |
| *Omega-3 Fatty Acids* | | |
| fish oil (OTC) | | 3–6 g per day |
| | Lovaza (Rx) | 4 g per day |
| *Combinations* | | |
| atorvastatin/amlodipine | Caduet | PO daily; dose varies with response |
| ezetimibe/simvastatin | Vytorin | PO daily evening; dose varies with response |
| lovastatin/niacin | Advicor | PO daily bedtime with food; dose varies with response |

*Note:* Other antilipemic agents are available. Some reduce triglycerides as well.

## PATIENT EDUCATION

Patients on antilipemic therapy should be instructed regarding:

Continuing diet (low-fat, low-cholesterol) and aerobic exercise

Taking the medicine with meals to reduce GI upset

Reporting side effects to the physician immediately, *especially muscle pain, tenderness, weakness, dark-stained urine, or bleeding*

With cholestyramine, the importance of a high-fiber diet and/or a stool softener, fat-soluble vitamin and folic acid supplements, and not taking other medication within 4h

Expecting facial flushing with niacin (unless extended-release formula is used)

Taking most statins in the evening (the body synthesizes most cholesterol at night)

*Avoiding grapefruit juice* while taking statins; adverse effects are potentiated

Giving their health care provider a list of all the medicines, herbs, nonprescription drugs, or dietary supplements they are taking so that potential interactions can be identified

The importance of initial liver function tests

If all the other factors remain the same, the medication will probably need to be taken throughout the patient's lifetime. Sometimes diet and exercise will eliminate the need.

# ANTITHROMBOTIC AGENTS

Blood has the ability to flow freely through blood vessels yet clot when the need arises. Normal hemostasis or blood coagulation involves the formation of a fibrin clot or thrombus so a minor cut would not cause us to bleed profusely. However, inappropriate thrombus formation can be caused by vessel-wall injury, circulatory stasis, increased blood coagulability, immobilization, obesity, cigarette smoking, medication therapy, and other factors. The inappropriate thrombus formation or clot can dislodge and travel through the bloodstream (thromboembolism or TE) where it can fully or partially obstruct blood flow, leading to tissue damage. Antithrombotic agents, which interfere with or prevent thrombosis or blood coagulation, include anticoagulants, platelet inhibitors, and thrombolytics.

## Anticoagulants

Anticoagulants prevent the formation of the fibrin clot by interfering with one of the steps leading to fibrin formation. They are divided into two general groups: oral (coumarin derivatives and the new oral anticoagulants) and injectable (heparins). The action of these two classes is quite different. However, their purpose is the same: to prevent the formation of clots or decrease the extension of existing clots in such conditions as venous thrombosis, stroke, pulmonary embolism, and coronary artery occlusion. Also, many patients with artificial heart valves, mitral valve disease, or chronic atrial fibrillation, or postsurgical patients (cardiac bypass, vascular surgery, and hip or knee replacement) receive anticoagulants to prevent embolism or thrombosis. Patients on anticoagulants, especially older patients, should be constantly observed for *bleeding complications*, such as cerebrovascular accidents (CVAs). The coumarin derivatives (warfarin) and heparin do not dissolve existing clots; they only interfere with the coagulation process preventing clot formation and/or propagation.

# Warfarin

Warfarin (Coumadin) is administered *orally* (it is also available as an injectable preparation, which is rarely used). This medicine alters the synthesis of blood coagulation factors in the liver by interfering with the action of vitamin K. The *antidote for serious bleeding complications during warfarin therapy is prothrombin complex concentrate or fresh frozen plasma and vitamin K.* The action of warfarin is slower than that of heparin; therefore, warfarin is generally used as follow-up for long-term anticoagulant therapy, although warfarin may be started at the same time as heparin.

The most commonly used laboratory method of monitoring therapy with warfarin is the International Normalized Ratio (INR). The INR serves as a guide in determining the dosage.

Interactions of warfarin with *many* drugs have been reported. Concurrent administration of any other drug should be investigated, and the following drugs should be *avoided* if possible. Some of the drugs that may *increase* response to warfarin include:

Anabolic steroids

Alcohol (acute intoxication)

Proton pump inhibitors

All NSAIDs, including aspirin; thrombolytics

Tricyclic antidepressants; SSRIs

Thyroid drugs

Amiodarone, propafenone, and quinidine

Many anti-infective agents

Many antilipemic agents

Acetaminophen (large daily doses or long duration)

Grapefruit juice, fish oil, vitamin E, many herbal supplements

Some of the drugs that may *decrease* response to warfarin include:

Alcohol (chronic alcoholism)

Barbiturates

Estrogen (including oral contraceptives)

Antiretroviral protease inhibitors

There are many other interactions with warfarin. Always check before administering any other medicine.

## New Oral Anticoagulants

Although warfarin was the mainstay of oral anticoagulation therapy for over 50 years, its significant limitations and interactions have led to the research and development for acceptable alternatives. In October 2009, dabigatran (Pradaxa) was the first oral anticoagulant (direct thrombin inhibitor) to be approved by the FDA in more than half a century. This was followed by the approval of two more oral anticoagulants (factor Xa inhibitors)—rivaroxaban (Xarelto) and most recently apixaban (Eliquis).

Compared to warfarin, the new oral anticoagulants have a rapid onset and predictable anticoagulant effects and fewer food and drug interactions; routine laboratory monitoring is not required.

However, anticoagulant effects cannot be monitored with standard laboratory testing, and there is currently no reversal agent in case of uncontrolled major bleeding or the need for emergency surgery (although some are in early clinical trials).

Dabigatran, rivaroxaban, and apixaban are all indicated for reducing the risk of stroke and systemic embolism in patients with nonvalvular atrial fibrillation. Rivaroxaban is also indicated for venous thromboembolism prevention, post-hip or -knee replacement, and DVT/PE treatment or prevention of recurrence.

## Heparin and Low-Molecular-Weight Heparins

There are two types of heparin: the standard or unfractionated type (UFH) and the low-molecular-weight heparins (LMWHs).

Heparin is not absorbed from the GI tract, and the standard type (UFH) must be administered *intravenously* or *subcutaneously*. The LMWH type is usually only administered subcutaneously but may be given IV as well. Heparin acts on thrombin, inhibiting the action of fibrin in clot formation. The *antidote for serious bleeding complications during heparin therapy is protamine sulfate.* When administered IV, the action of heparin is immediate. A *dilute flushing* solution of heparin is also used to maintain the patency of indwelling venipuncture devices used to obtain blood specimens and of catheters used for arterial access (arterial lines). *Be sure to check that it is a dilute flushing solution before injection, and not full-strength heparin.* However, 0.9% sodium chloride (normal saline) injection alone is used to flush *peripheral* venipuncture devices, for example PRN adapters. Heparin is *not* normally used to flush these devices because of possible drug incompatibilities and laboratory test interferences.

The LMWHs include enoxaparin (Lovenox) and dalteparin (Fragmin). When administered subcutaneously, monitoring of anticoagulant effect is not necessary, but periodic complete blood counts (CBCs), stool occult blood tests, and platelet counts are recommended during treatment.

Unlike UFH, in the case of clinically significant bleeding, no agent fully reverses the activity of the LMWHs, although protamine has some activity and should be given for life-threatening bleeding along with packed red blood cells and fresh frozen plasma transfusions if indicated. Fondaparinux (Arixtra), a closely related pentasaccharide, is not generally classified as an LMWH (although often discussed with the same). It is an indirect clotting factor Xa inhibitor and lacks a specific antidote in the event of excessive anticoagulation.

Enoxaparin was the first LMWH to be approved in the United States. It is currently approved for the prevention of deep vein thrombosis (DVT) in patients undergoing hip or knee replacement or abdominal surgery, for the treatment of unstable angina and ST-elevation myocardial infarction (STEMI), and for the in-patient treatment of acute DVT and pulmonary embolism (PE). It is also used in the outpatient treatment of acute DVT not associated with pulmonary embolism and is combined with warfarin (until INR reaches 2–3).

When heparin is administered subcutaneously, especially if the patient is discharged and the medication will be administered at home, be sure to stress *patient education.* See also Chapter 9, "Administration by the Parenteral Route."

Measurement of the activated partial thromboplastin time (aPTT) is the most common laboratory test for monitoring heparin therapy. When long-term anticoagulant therapy is begun with warfarin, there is a short-term overlap period in which both heparin and warfarin are administered concurrently.

Interactions of all anticoagulants with other anticoagulants, for example aspirin and NSAIDs, platelet inhibitors, and fish oil, or with thrombolytic agents, for example alteplase (tPA), may increase the risk of hemorrhage.

Side effects of all anticoagulants can include:

- Major hemorrhage
- Thrombocytopenia
- Minor bleeding (e.g., petechiae, nosebleed, and bruising)
- Blood in the urine (hematuria) or stools (melena)
- Osteoporosis with long-term heparin use (less with the LMWHs; none with the other agents)

Precautions or contraindications for anticoagulants apply to:

GI disorders and ulceration of GI tract

Hepatic and renal dysfunction

Blood dyscrasias

Pregnancy (heparin can be used with caution as it does not cross the placenta)

Stroke (may increase the risk of fatal cerebral hemorrhage after stroke)

Patients with prosthetic heart valves (with the new oral anticoagulants)

Lumbar puncture and epidural anesthesia (could result in paralysis)

See Table 25-5 for a summary of the anticoagulants.

**TABLE 25-5** Anticoagulants

| GENERIC NAME | TRADE NAME | DOSAGE |
|---|---|---|
| **Anticoagulants, Oral** | | |
| *Coumarin Derivative* | | |
| Warfarin | Coumadin, Jantoven | PO dose varies, based on PT/INR results |
| *Factor Xa Inhibitors* | | |
| apixaban | Eliquis | PO 2.5–5 mg two times per day |
| rivaroxaban | Xarelto | PO 20 mg one time daily with P.M. meal (stroke prevention) |
| | | PO 15 mg two times daily for three weeks, and then 20 mg one time daily with food (DVT/PE treatment or prevention) |
| | | PO 10 mg once daily for 35 days (post-hip replacement) |
| | | PO 10 mg one time daily for 12 days (post-knee replacement) |
| *Thrombin Inhibitor* | | |
| dabigatran | Pradaxa | PO 150 mg two times daily (75 mg for CrCl 15–30); store in original container only up to four months |
| **Anticoagulants, Injectable** | | |
| *Unfractionated Heparin* | | |
| Heparin | | IV, subcu dose varies |
| *Low-Molecular-Weight Heparins* | | |
| Dalteparin | Fragmin | Subcu, in fixed or body-weight-adjusted doses one to two times daily |
| Enoxaparin | Lovenox | One to two times daily subcu dose and duration varies; reduce dose for CrCl <30 mL/min |
| *Factor Xa Inhibitor* | | |
| Fondaparinux | Arixtra | Daily subcutaneous dose varies; closely related to the LMWHs |

**Note:** This is a representative sample; many other products are available.

## Platelet Inhibitor Therapy

Antiplatelet agents inhibit the aggregation (clumping) and release of thromboplastin from the platelets to begin the clotting process. Platelet inhibitors utilize a variety of mechanisms to interfere with activation pathways to prevent platelet clumping and are given as prophylactic therapy or as secondary prevention in patients with a history of recent stroke, recent MI, or established peripheral vascular disease. They are also used in the pharmacologic management of post-acute coronary syndrome (ACS), a spectrum of clinical conditions ranging from unstable angina to acute myocardial infarction, with or without ST-segment elevation. Platelet inhibitors are also used prior to and following percutaneous coronary intervention (PCI) with coronary stenting to prevent stent thrombosis.

# PATIENT EDUCATION

It is very *important* that patients on anticoagulant therapy be instructed regarding:

Reading the FDA-approved Medication Guide dispensed with the oral anticoagulants

Importance of compliance with taking medications as prescribed and required laboratory monitoring (if any)

The fact that this medication does not dissolve clots and that it decreases the clotting ability of the blood and helps prevent the formation of harmful blood clots in the blood vessels and heart

Taking the medication as prescribed at the same time every day

Not changing brands of the medication without the physician's approval

Avoiding eating large amounts of grapefruit or drinking grapefruit juice or cranberry juice

Avoiding shots such as flu shots, shingle vaccine, and pneumonia vaccine (Talk with your health care provider before getting shots.)

Avoiding activities and contact sports that may cause injury, cuts, or bruises

Using a soft toothbrush and an electric razor to shave to prevent cuts

Always wearing closed-toe shoes

Using a night light to prevent falls

Immediately reporting unusual bleeding, bruising, brown spots, or blood-tinged secretions, injury, trauma, dizziness, abdominal pain or swelling, back pain, headaches, and joint pain and swelling to their physician

If prescribed, carrying vitamin K for emergency use

Using a reliable birth control method

Reporting allergic reactions such as skin rash to their physicians

Avoiding smoking, the use of alcohol, and over-the-counter medications

Wearing identifications and alerts at all times

Keeping all follow-up appointments with their physician for laboratory work and for needed dosage changes

***Note:*** Large amounts of vitamin K–rich foods can counteract warfarin therapy. Be consistent with your intake of foods high in vitamin K such as asparagus, broccoli, cabbage, Brussels sprouts, spinach, turnips, dried fruits, bananas, potatoes, peaches, and tomatoes to ensure a stable INR.

In addition to drug therapy, patients should be educated on modifying risk factors for CHD and stroke, that is, abstinence from all forms of tobacco, weight control, low-fat and low-cholesterol diet, and aerobic exercise on a regular basis.

## Dipyridamole (Persantine)

Dipyridamole (Persantine) is a non-nitrate coronary vasodilator that inhibits platelet aggregation. When used alone, it is ineffective as an antithrombotic for patients with AMI, DVT, or transient ischemic attacks (TIAs) and therefore must be combined with other anticoagulant drugs. Dipyridamole is used in combination with aspirin in the prevention of ischemic stroke.

Side effects of dipyridamole, usually transient, can include:

Headache, dizziness, and weakness

Nausea, vomiting, and diarrhea

Flushing and rash

Caution with older adults (more susceptible to orthostatic hypotension).

A combination of low-dose aspirin with extended-release dipyridamole (Aggrenox) is approved for stroke prophylaxis. Most adverse effects are mild and similar to those with either agent alone.

## Aspirin

Because of its ability to inhibit platelet aggregation, aspirin has been studied extensively for use in the prevention of thrombosis. Aspirin therapy, usually 75–325 mg daily, has been used after myocardial infarction or recurrent TIAs to reduce the risk of recurrence. Aspirin has also been used to reduce the risk of myocardial infarction in patients with unstable angina.

Aspirin therapy is not recommended for low-risk patients because of an increased risk of hemorrhagic stroke associated with long-term aspirin therapy. Patients should be instructed not to start aspirin therapy without consulting a physician first. Because of *gastric irritation*, aspirin should be administered with food or milk. Film-coated tablets, enteric-coated tablets, and buffered aspirin preparations are available to reduce gastric irritation. Aspirin is *contraindicated* for anyone with bleeding disorders. See Chapter 19 for a description of other side effects, precautions or contraindications, and interactions.

## Adenosine Diphosphate (ADP) Receptor Antagonists

ADP receptor antagonists block the activation of the platelet's receptor surface, thereby inhibiting platelet activation. Clopidogrel (Plavix) was the first agent approved in this class. It is used to reduce atherosclerotic events (myocardial infarction, stroke, and vascular death) in patients with a history of recent stroke, recent MI, or established peripheral vascular disease.

Clopidogrel is also used in combination with aspirin to prevent thrombosis of stents that are used to prop open diseased coronary arteries. Prasugrel (Effient) is a more potent antiplatelet agent with no clinically significant drug interactions identified to date.

The newest agent in this class, ticagrelor (Brilinta), is the first reversible oral ADP receptor antagonist. Its quicker onset of antiplatelet activity allows the platelet function to return to baseline quicker and may result in fewer coronary artery bypass surgery–related bleeding events in patients requiring emergent intervention. Ticagrelor's shorter half-life necessitates twice-daily dosing compared with once-daily dosing of clopidogrel and prasugrel. Ticagrelor is contraindicated in severe hepatic impairment.

All ADP receptor antagonists are **contraindicated** in patients with active pathological bleeding (such as peptic ulcer) or a history of intracranial hemorrhage. **Interactions** of all platelet inhibitors with other anticoagulants, for example aspirin and NSAIDs, other platelet inhibitors, or thrombolytic agents, may increase the risk of bleeding.

The use of certain PPIs (esomeprazole, omeprazole, including Prilosec OTC), azole antifungals, most macrolide antibiotics (except azithromycin), certain SSRIs (fluoxetine, fluvoxamine), and HIV NNRTIs may make clopidogrel less effective by inhibiting the enzyme that converts clopidogrel to the active form of the drug. The plasma concentrations of ticagrelor may be elevated by azole antifungals, HIV protease inhibitors, and some macrolide antibiotics; they may be reduced by carbamazepine, phenobarbital, phenytoin, and rifampin. Ticagrelor can increase digoxin concentrations (monitor levels) and increase lovastatin and simvastatin concentrations (avoid doses > 40 mg).

# THROMBOLYTIC AGENTS

The body maintains a process to dissolve clots (fibrinolysis) after they have formed. Tissue plasminogen activator (t-PA) is a natural peptide that initiates fibrinolysis. Thrombolytic agents actually dissolve and liquefy the fibrin of the existing clot. Thrombolytic drugs (e.g., reteplase and alteplase) potentiate t-PA, resulting in clot dissolution, reperfusion of organs, and restoration of blood flow to tissues.

Thrombolytic agents, given IV, reduce mortality when used as early as possible but within the first 12h after the onset of acute STEMI. Alteplase is also used to treat acute ischemic stroke (within 3 to 4.5h of the onset of stroke symptoms) and acute pulmonary embolism. Administered in an ER or ICU setting, close monitoring of hemodynamics and vital signs is generally considered standard with thrombolytic therapy, particularly during the initial 24–48h.

Intracranial hemorrhage is the most serious complication of thrombolytic therapy, but bleeding can occur at any site in the body. Bleeding occurs most commonly at access sites such as catheter insertion sites or venipuncture sites. Patients with preexisting coagulation problems, uncontrolled hypertension, severe chronic heart failure, and recent stroke are at the highest risk for developing bleeding complications during thrombolytic therapy.

Hemorrhage can result from concomitant therapy with heparin or other platelet-aggregation inhibitors. If severe bleeding occurs during therapy, the drug should be discontinued promptly. Rapid coronary lysis can result in the development of arrhythmias; however, they are generally transient in nature.

# HEMATOPOIETIC AGENTS

Hematopoiesis is the formation, differentiation, and maturation of blood cells into specific cell lines. Hematopoietic agents to be discussed here include erythropoiesis-stimulating agents and the colony-stimulating factors. All hematopoietic agents are products of recombinant technology.

# Erythropoiesis-Stimulating Agents

The erythropoiesis-stimulating agents (ESAs) such as epoetin alfa (Epogen or Procrit) are responsible for the regulation of the production and development of blood cells, normally in the bone marrow. Epoetin alfa stimulates the bone marrow to produce more red blood cells and is approved for the treatment of anemia in chronic renal failure, HIV infection, and anemia associated with chemotherapy. It also reduces the need for blood transfusions in anemic patients scheduled to undergo certain kinds of surgery. Darbepoetin alfa (Aranesp) is a *second-generation* agent that is dosed less frequently than epoetin alfa.

Before initiating ESA therapy, supplemental iron (folic acid, and/or vitamin $B_{12}$ if necessary) is usually needed because adequate iron stores are necessary to incorporate iron into hemoglobin. Treatment of iron deficiency by regular use of iron improves erythropoiesis and response to ESA therapy. As of March 2010, prescribers and hospitals must enroll in and comply with the ESA APPRISE Oncology Program to prescribe and/or dispense epoetin alfa to patients with cancer. Recently, the FDA once again updated safety information in the black box warning regarding the use of ESAs: Use the lowest dose possible to gradually increase the hemoglobin (Hgb) concentration to avoid the need for transfusion.

Side effects of epoetin alfa (Epogen) include:

- Hypertension (especially in dialysis patients)
- Flu-like symptoms
  - GI effects
  - Rash
  - Chest pain
- Increased mortality, MI, stroke, thrombosis of vascular access, venous thromboembolic events, and increased risk of tumor progression or recurrence

# Colony Stimulating Factors (CSFs)

A granulocyte colony-stimulating factor (G-CSF), filgrastim (Neupogen) is involved in the regulation and production of neutrophils in response to host defense needs. It lessens the severity of myelosuppression in patients with cancer and has allowed chemotherapy dose intensification or maintenance of dose intensity. Use with caution in patients with sickle cell disorders.

Side effects of filgrastim include:

  Bone pain (common)

  Headache

  Dermatological reactions

See Table 25-6 for a summary of platelet inhibitors, thrombolytic agents, and hematopoetic agents.

**TABLE 25-6** Platelet Inhibitors, Thrombolytic Agents, and Hematopoetic Agents

| GENERIC NAME | TRADE NAME | DOSAGE |
|---|---|---|
| **Platelet Inhibitors** | | |
| aspirin | Ecotrin, Ascriptin, others | 75–325 mg PO daily |
| dipyridamole | Persantine | 75–100 mg PO four times per day with warfarin or aspirin depending on indication |
| dipyridamole with aspirin | Aggrenox | 1 cap PO BID |
| *ADP Receptor Antagonists* | | |
| clopidogrel | Plavix | 75 mg PO daily with or without food; 300 mg loading dose in ACS, usually with low-dose aspirin |
| prasugrel | Effient | 60 mg PO loading dose and then 10 mg daily (5 mg if < 60 kg) with aspirin for ACS managed with PCI |
| ticagrelor | Brilinta | 180 mg PO loading dose and then 90 mg twice daily with aspirin (100 mg max) for ACS |
| **Thrombolytic Agents** | | |
| alteplase, tPA | Activase | IV bolus and then IV infusion |
| | Cathflo Activase | 2 mg injection one time (MR in 2 h) for IV catheter occlusions |
| reteplase, r-PA | Retavase | IV bolus two times (30 min apart) |
| tenecteplase, TNK-tPA | TNKase | Rapid IV bolus |
| **Hematopoetic Agents** | | |
| *ESAs* | | |
| darbepoetin alfa | Aranesp | IV, subcutaneous dose varies |
| epoetin alfa | Epogen, Procrit | IV, subcutaneous dose varies |
| *CSFs* | | |
| filgrastim, G-CSF | Neupogen | IV, subcutaneous dose varies |

**Note:** This is a representative sample; many other products are available.

# CASE STUDY A

## CARDIOVASCULAR DRUGS

Isaac Doniego, a 77-year-old widower with heart failure, has been treated successfully with a combination of ACE inhibitors and diuretics. However, his symptoms worsen and became life threatening despite pharmacologic treatment, so he is hospitalized for evaluation and stabilization on a cardiac glycoside.

1. How will the cardiac glycoside act to lessen Isaac's heart failure?
   a. By increasing his heart rate
   b. By increasing the force of cardiac contraction
   c. By increasing his oxygen utilization
   d. By suppressing possible cardiac arrhythmias

2. What type of cardiac glycoside is Isaac's physician most likely to prescribe?
   a. Synthetic adenosine            c. Digitalis product
   b. Lidocaine or a related drug     d. Thiazide

3. Isaac's physician alerts him that cardiac glycosides should be avoided if he has which of the following conditions?
   a. Hyperthyroidism               c. Hypermagnesemia
   b. Hyperkalemia                  d. Impaired renal function

4. Isaac should be advised to avoid certain medications because they can potentiate digoxin toxicity. Which of the following are in this category?
   a. Cholestyramine, neomycin, and rifampin
   b. Diuretics, calcium, and corticosteroids
   c. Macrolides and antiarrhythmics
   d. Adrenergics

5. Isaac should be cautioned about taking antacids because of the risk of:
   a. Reduced absorption of digoxin
   b. Arrhythmia
   c. Digoxin toxicity
   d. Increased force of cardiac contraction

# CASE STUDY B

## CARDIOVASCULAR DRUGS

Dianna Whitfield, a 37-year-old African-American, has been diagnosed with hypertension. Her physician discusses various options for pharmacologic treatment.

1. What class of drugs is Dianna's physician most likely to prescribe first?
   a. Thiazides
   b. Beta-blockers
   c. ACE inhibitors
   d. Calcium channel blockers

2. What antihypertensives are known to be *more* effective in African-Americans and older adults?
   a. Thiazides
   b. Angiotensin receptor blockers
   c. Nonthiazide diuretics
   d. Calcium channel blockers

3. What antihypertensives are known to be *less* effective in African-Americans than in other groups?
   a. Beta-adrenergic blockers
   b. Antiadrenergics
   c. ACE inhibitors
   d. Peripheral vasodilators

4. Dianna also has lupus. What class of antihypertensive should be avoided?
   a. Beta-adrenergic blockers
   b. Antiadrenergics
   c. ACE inhibitors
   d. Thiazides

5. Suppose Dianna is pregnant and experiences preeclampsia. Under this circumstance, the antihypertensive of choice would likely be:
   a. Chlorthalidone
   b. Hydralazine
   c. Losartan
   d. Enalapril

# CHAPTER REVIEW QUIZ

Match the medication in the first column with the condition in the second column that it is used to treat. Conditions may be used more than once.

**Medication**

1. _____ isosorbide
2. _____ Zetia
3. _____ Lovenox
4. _____ Cardizem
5. _____ Zocor
6. _____ Plavix
7. _____ Crestor
8. _____ hydralazine
9. _____ quinidine
10. _____ procainamide

**Classification**

**a.** Elevated cholesterol

**b.** Hypertension

**c.** Angina

**d.** Pulmonary emboli

**e.** Cardiac arrhythmia

**f.** Stroke prevention (platelet inhibitor)

**Choose the correct answer.**

11. Why is digoxin the only cardiac glycoside and digitalis product still marketed for clinical use?

    **a.** It is safe at higher doses.

    **b.** It is effective on cardiac arrhythmias.

    **c.** It is slow acting.

    **d.** It can be administered orally and parenterally.

12. About what percentage of adults in the United States are considered to have prehypertension?

    **a.** 27%

    **b.** 37%

    **c.** 47%

    **d.** 57%

13. Digoxin toxicity can usually be treated sufficiently by:

    **a.** Discontinuing digoxin

    **b.** Administering atropine

    **c.** Treating potassium and magnesium disturbances

    **d.** Administering digoxin-specific Fab fragments

14. Fibrillation refers to:

    **a.** Rapid heartbeat

    **b.** Irregular heart beat

    **c.** Slow heart beat

    **d.** Insufficient heart beat

15. Most drugs given to counteract arrhythmias have the potential for:

    **a.** Causing hypertensive crisis

    **b.** Deranging calcium levels

    **c.** Slowing the heart rate

    **d.** Increasing glucose metabolism

16. Which of the following is especially important to monitor in patients receiving antiarrhythmic drugs?

    **a.** Electrolytes

    **b.** Glucose

    **c.** Platelets

    **d.** Lipids

17. Which of the following has been widely accepted as the most effective treatment for patients with life-threatening ventricular tachycardia or fibrillation?

    a. Insertion of an AICD                    c. Adenosine
    b. Amiodarone                              d. Propranolol

18. Inhibition of ACE lowers blood pressure by:

    a. Decreasing cardiac output               c. Decreasing vasoconstriction
    b. Increasing cardiac output               d. Increasing vasoconstriction

19. Side effects from beta-blockers are most common in:

    a. Patients of age 50 or younger
    b. Patients receiving IV administration of the drug
    c. Patients with pre-existing arrhythmia
    d. Patients who suffer from migraines

20. Coronary vasodilators are used for the:

    a. Treatment of hypotension
    b. Reduction of intracranial pressure
    c. Prevention of tachycardia and resulting syncope
    d. Treatment of angina

21. Increased risk of new-onset diabetes mellitus is most associated with high doses of:

    a. Statins                                 c. Calcium channel blockers
    b. Cardiac glycosides                      d. Bile acid sequestrants

22. Which drug is *least* effective in reducing the mortality associated with heart failure?

    a. Metoprolol                              c. Bisoprolol
    b. Atenolol                                d. Carvedilol

23. What is one purpose of International Normalized Ratio (INR) monitoring?

    a. To monitor warfarin therapy
    b. To monitor kidney function for persons on antilipemics
    c. To determine the need for pharmacologic treatment of angina
    d. To determine the effectiveness of antihypertensives

24. How are low-molecular-weight heparins usually administered?

    a. Orally                                  c. Subcutaneously
    b. Sublingually                            d. As a skin patch

25. What is an advantage of the new oral anticoagulants?

    a. Slow onset for long-term therapy
    b. Fewer food and drug interactions
    c. Ability to monitor with standard laboratory equipment
    d. Availability of numerous reversal agents

---

**STUDY**GUIDE                     **Online Resources**LINK

**P R A C T I C E**

Complete Chapter 25                • PowerPoint presentations